Make Peace With Painful Memories

Learn How to Forgive When You Cannot Forget: Tips on Creating a Beautiful Life

Dawn Hazel

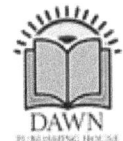

© Copyright 2022 - All rights reserved.

The content contained within this book may not be reproduced, duplicated or transmitted without direct written permission from the author or the publisher.

Under no circumstances will any blame or legal responsibility be held against the publisher, or author, for any damages, reparation, or monetary loss due to the information contained within this book, either directly or indirectly.

Legal Notice:

This book is copyright protected. It is only for personal use. You cannot amend, distribute, sell, use, quote or paraphrase any part, or the content within this book, without the consent of the author or publisher.

Disclaimer Notice:

Please note the information contained within this document is for educational and entertainment purposes only. All effort has been executed to present accurate, up to date, reliable, complete information. No warranties of any kind are declared or implied. Readers acknowledge that the author is not engaged in the rendering of legal, financial, medical or professional advice. The content within this book has been derived from various sources. Please consult a licensed professional before attempting any techniques outlined in this book.

By reading this document, the reader agrees that under no circumstances is the author responsible for any losses, direct or indirect, that are incurred as a result of the use of the information contained within this document, including, but not limited to, errors, omissions, or inaccuracies.

Table of Contents

INTRODUCTION 1

    INVITATION TO JOIN THE FORGIVENESS CRUISE 2
        A Word From Your Captain 2
        Preparing to Capture the Sunset 3
        A Glimpse at the All-Inclusive Itinerary 4
    ALL ABOARD 4

CHAPTER 1: RESIDUAL EMOTIONAL BAGGAGE: THE LINGERING EFFECTS OF THE PAIN CAUSED BY HEARTACHE 7

    UNDERSTANDING THE NEGATIVE EFFECTS OF EMOTIONAL BAGGAGE 8
        Sorting Through Luggage 9
    HEALTH: WEIGHED DOWN UNDER THE BAGGAGE 10
        Cortisol: The Stress Regulator 12

CHAPTER 2: HOW TO GET THROUGH THE PAIN, HEARTACHE, AND ANGER ASSOCIATED WITH TRAUMA 17

    DO WHAT IS RIGHT FOR YOU, AND NOT FOR ANYONE ELSE 19
        Identifying Physical and Emotional Symptoms of Traumatic Stress 20
    RECOVERING FROM TRAUMA MAY BE EASIER THAN YOU THINK 23
        Small Steps in the Right Direction 25

CHAPTER 3: WHY YOU SHOULD CUT YOURSELF SOME SLACK 29

    THE EFFECTS OF DEALING WITH PAIN 30
        Compartmentalizing the Contents of the Emotional Baggage 31
        How to Limit Excess Luggage 32

CHAPTER 4: LEARNING HOW TO FORGIVE 37

    THE INS AND OUTS: UNDERSTANDING AND BENEFITS OF FORGIVENESS 38
        Understanding Forgiveness 39
        Benefits of Forgiveness 41
    THE BLUEPRINTS FOR YOUR HEALING PROCESS 42
        Preparation 43
        Identifying the Pain 43
        What Is the Purpose of Suffering? 45

CHAPTER 5: ESTABLISHING BOUNDARIES TO PROTECT YOURSELF 47

    UNDERSTANDING THE PURPOSE OF BOUNDARIES 48

    The Importance of Boundaries 49
    The Different Types of Boundaries You Need to Establish 50
  THE BENEFITS OF BOUNDARIES 54
    Setting Yourself up for Success 54

CHAPTER 6: LEARNING HOW TO LET GO OF GRUDGES 57

  SIGNS THAT YOU ARE HOLDING A GRUDGE 58
    Inspecting the Root of Grudges 60
    Inspecting Our Toxic Dumpsites 61
  MOVING ON AND LETTING GO 63
    Journaling 64
    Changing Perspective 65
    Roundup 65

CHAPTER 7: UTILIZING ALTERNATIVE PRACTICES TO EASE THE JOURNEY TO FORGIVENESS 67

  SELF-HEALING TECHNIQUES THAT WORK 68
    Forgiveness Technique: An Ancient Hawaiian Mantra 69
    Forgiveness Technique: Meditation 71

CHAPTER 8: I THOUGHT GOD WOULD PROTECT ME FROM PAIN AND SUFFERING 77

  CROSSING THE BRIDGE OF RELIGION 78
    Why Does God Allow Suffering? 79
    What Is the Purpose of Suffering? 81

CHAPTER 9: START OVER BY REDISCOVERING RELIGION 87

  FINDING THE RIGHT PATH 88
    Every Journey Starts Somewhere 90
    Helping You Overcome Obstacles 91
    Love, Hope, and Faith 94

CONCLUSION 97

  IT'S OKAY NOT TO BE OKAY 97
    Hearty Reassurances 98
    Until We Meet Again: Thank you, and See You Later 99

REFERENCES 101

  IMAGE REFERENCES 106

Introduction

To forgive is the highest, most beautiful form of love. In return, you will receive untold peace and happiness. —Robert Muller

- Do you feel as if you are trapped in an invisible cage that you can't break out of?

- What is preventing you from breaking out of that cage?

- How are you going to break free from the cage that is holding you hostage?

I believe that everyone has experienced this invisible cage I have alluded to at some stage during their lives. Many may not want to admit that they are—or have been—held hostage in these cages once, twice, or multiple times. I want to tell you a little secret. Come closer. Don't be afraid. A little bit closer. You don't have to be afraid or embarrassed to admit that you are, or have been, a resident of this invisible cage. Whatever has happened to trap you in your invisible cage has no power over you in the real world. You can't change what happened in the past, but you can shape your future.

Don't give these invisible cages the power to suck the life out of you. Don't allow them to fill you with fear. No one has the right to weigh you down by taking away your right to happiness. Yes, I know that it is easier said than done. You may even be rolling your eyes and thinking, *What does she know?* I have told you that everyone is, and has been, in this position at some point during their lives. It is not an uncommon occurrence, and everyone—regardless of age, gender, religion or spirituality, or ethnicity—has been where you are.

Invitation to Join the Forgiveness Cruise

You are cordially invited to join on the Forgiveness Cruise. I am the captain, deckhand, engineer, entertainer, resident lifeguard, chaplain, and the voice of reason. I take my responsibilities seriously, because I want all passengers to feel comfortable at all times. You may experience some adverse weather conditions as we sail off to capture the elusive sunset. This cruise liner will be dropping anchor at 10 different ports. Each port we dock at will take you on a sightseeing expedition that will attempt to help you break free from your invisible cage.

A Word From Your Captain

You will not be forced to do anything you are not comfortable with. You are in control at all times. This cruise is all about you, and what is beneficial for your health and mental well-being. This cruise will provide you with a safe space that is free of judgment, condemnation, and bullying. You are the priority, and you are going to learn how to prioritize the most important person in your life—YOU! Who is going to prioritize you when you are cowering in a corner because you are afraid of painful or hurtful memories? You are going to learn how to obliterate that invisible cage, put yourself on a podium, and take back what has been taken from you. It is time for you to shine brighter than all the stars in the night sky.

The Forgiveness Cruise is not going to be like any other cruise you may or may not have been on or read about. How many hands do you need to count the number of times someone has told you to, "forgive and forget," something that has happened to you? I would be a multimillionaire, sipping piña coladas on a tropical island, if I got a dollar for every time someone told me to, "forgive and forget," someone or something. Have the people who tell others to forgive and forget never experienced holding onto grudges or bitterness? Have they never experienced the pain inflicted on them by the wrongdoing of others? I refuse to speculate on what other people have been, or are going, through. It is not my place to pass judgment on other people's situations or circumstances. I know and understand the frustration of being told what to do, and how to deal, with something. Some may call it unsolicited advice, and others may call it interfering where it is not necessary.

This book is not going to tell you what you should be doing or should not be doing. Life is all about choices. There is not enough bubble wrap and cotton wool in the world to protect everyone from the knocks that they will encounter during their lifetime. New parents are not given manuals when their babies are born. They have to rely on their instincts, and the love they have for their newborns. You can protect (or try to) your baby and toddler as much as possible, but they will eventually fall and bump their heads, split a lip, or take a tumble. What happens when you grow up? What happens when you are an adult? You will grow up because it is part of life. You cannot hide behind your parents. You will encounter moments during your lifetime where you will experience pain, anguish, and defeat. You will be filled with anger, rage, hatred, or fear because you believed that you were protected from life experiences.

Preparing to Capture the Sunset

Your journey through life will include more bumps, split lips, and tumbles that you could never have foreseen. You will encounter moments during your lifetime where you will experience the wash, rinse, and spin cycle on repeat. This book is going to help you navigate your way through some of those difficult moments that hold you hostage. The invisible cage that I have mentioned is built up of anger, rage, hatred, fear, love, sadness, regret, and everything that negatively affects your mind, body, and soul. I am not going to set unrealistic expectations. I am not going to tell you what you must do to break through your invisible cage. I will be sharing tried and tested tools based on what I have gathered during my research.

This book is about forgiving those who have purposefully caused you pain and suffering. You may even learn about seeking forgiveness against someone *you* have hurt. This is a journey that is going to take time, and lots of patience. No one is going to expect you to move a mountain. You will learn the essential tips and tricks that will help lighten the load that is weighing you down. You are going to resolve some of those unanswered questions that are bouncing around in your mind. You are going to learn how to find peace and happiness within yourself. I may be the captain of the Forgiveness Cruise, but you are the VIP passenger. And as the VIP passenger, you get to enjoy the perks of immersing yourself in the soft lull of the ocean when the storm passes.

A Glimpse at the All-Inclusive Itinerary

As I mentioned, being a VIP passenger onboard the Forgiveness Cruise comes with perks. One of the most important perks of being a VIP passenger is that you can take as many trips as you need or want for a lifetime. You will never be denied access once you purchase the all-inclusive Forgiveness Cruise package. You will receive unlimited private island tours. I would personally recommend the island tours, because they are tailor-made to suit any circumstance or situation you may be experiencing. Each of the tours will attempt to point you in a positive direction for you to understand, accept, and heal from whatever is holding you hostage. This is not a quick fix or surface solution to a problem that has been festering for a long time. This is merely giving you the stepping stones to help you find your way to a permanent solution.

All Aboard

Thank you for trusting me to be your captain on the Forgiveness Cruise. Your happiness, physical and mental health, and overall well-being are of utmost importance to everyone who cares about you. You may not see or feel it at this present moment in time, but you are the person that this world needs. I want everyone to know that you have destroyed the invisible cage that has been holding you hostage. I know that without saying anything, everyone will sense the peace that will radiate from you. I believe that you will encourage others to sparkle and shine themselves out of their invisible cages.

Safety Warning

This is a gentle reminder that you may not find or be open to the suggestions you will be presented with. You may resist any of the suggestions. You may even be angry at something you will read. I can promise you that there will be no attempts to control your mind, or bully you into doing something you are not ready to do. I know that you cannot snap your fingers, and your life will be changed. A more realistic approach would be slow and steady, where you set the pace. Take your time. Read this book more than once. This is *your* journey to finding freedom, it is not the journey of your mother, father, brother, sister, or best friend—it's your journey.

Let's Get Going

It is time to claim your cozy spot. You are free to test all the spots to find the right fit. Your kitchen will remain open for the duration of this cruise. Please be aware that you have options, such as scheduling a meal delivery through DoorDash. Ensure that you are stocked up on your beverage of choice, and snacks. Calories do not count on cruises, holidays, birthdays, or major milestones in your life. Sunscreen is optional, depending on the location of your cozy spot.

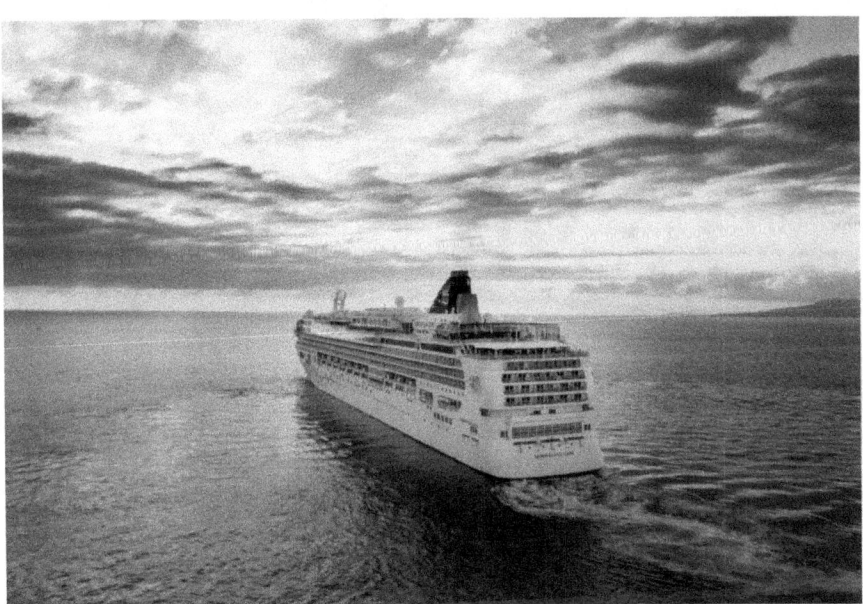

Chapter 1:

Residual Emotional Baggage: The Lingering Effects of the Pain Caused by Heartache

I get angry when I hear people say, "You'll get over it," "The pain won't last forever," "Stop looking for attention," or "Just forget about it." I have heard these nuggets of advice so many times that I can add them to my "tropical island" fund. I'd be able to buy the island and the surrounding ocean. I understand that friends and loved ones are trying to be helpful and encouraging. The problem is that no one knows the depth of pain someone is experiencing. Oh, you know that deep down they mean well. Some may say that they have been where you find yourself—but the reality is that not every situation is 100% the same. Everyone has their own battle that they are trying to wade through.

Yes, you're grateful for the support and encouragement. But you have to do what is best for you. Your road to healing and recovery is not paved with sunshine and roses. You don't know when you will ever be released from the clutches of pain, anger, or anxiety. You know that you have a safety net in those who love, care, and support you. You are also keenly aware that the safety net won't always offer the protection you require. This is the moment when you start realizing that any and all changes should begin with you.

I know that you are deathly afraid to take the next steps. Many have embarked on this journey of healing. Many are still on this journey. You reach a point in your life where you have had enough of everyone telling you how you should feel. I know that you want to break free from the chains that are restraining you. Did you know that you possess more power over your life than what you ever thought possible? I am a stranger telling you what you already know. You don't need me to confirm anything, because you are right where you need to be during this season of your life. I know that the future seems daunting, and you are hesitant to let go of your security blanket. The only piece of advice that I am going to offer you here and now is to tell you that it is time for you to believe in yourself.

Understanding the Negative Effects of Emotional Baggage

The island hopping commences right here and now. I am not going to make promises I can't keep. I am not going to offer any quick fixes or remedies. What I am going to do is ask you to keep an open mind for the duration of our journey together. Many people have, and continue to, navigate their way through the overgrown jungles that we call life. These jungles are relentless, and they prevent us from stepping out into a new world. We may say that we want to be free to live our lives. The intention to take that necessary step forward is genuine, until the moment of following through on the execution. The wheels start buckling, fall off, and roll as fast and as far as they possibly can. Everyone lives in a jungle where they feel safe. Is this the life you envisioned for yourself, though? This is not a multiple-choice question, and there is no right or wrong answer. This question cannot be answered on your behalf. You can cheat your way around it, but you are only cheating yourself. This question impacts the life of each person who answers it.

Let's turn the tables and ask a few more thought-provoking questions. Again, the questions have no right or wrong answers. No one will see or hear your answers unless you decide to share them. These questions are meant to help you assess where you are in your life, and whether you are ready to move out of the jungle where you have been hiding. Remember that you are the only one who can rifle through the baggage you have accumulated during all the seasons of your life.

- How are you feeling today?

- Did you wake up with a headache?

- Did you get out of bed feeling as if you would rather stay under the covers?

- Do you feel lethargic?

- Do you have a knot in your stomach?

- Are you staring out of the kitchen window with your cup of tea, and feeling the anger gurgling deep inside you?

- Are you feeling defeated, sad, angry, or afraid?

Sorting Through Luggage

Let's address the very large elephant-sized suitcase that you are carrying around. It is time to ask—not tell—you to lower the suitcase to the ground. Take a seat beside your suitcase and inhale, then exhale, a couple of well-deserved breaths. Open your mind and your heart, and be aware that you have choices. Relax in your safe zone while I rummage through the luggage that has been holding you hostage. My biggest wish for you is that you will experience the freedom of letting go of what is, and has been, weighing you down. It is time to get rid of the dirty laundry that has been dangled in front of your face, reminding you of whatever is threatening to suffocate you.

Your mental and physical health is of the utmost importance for you to operate and live a relatively normal life. You may argue and say that you are perfectly fine, and that you are not holding onto anything. I refer you to the questions I asked you in the previous section. Those questions are meant to make you think about where you are in your life journey. You don't have to answer those questions, but I do ask that you answer them honestly to yourself. I have experienced the side effects of lying to myself. And I am not the only one who has been lying, because it is easier to pretend that everything is sunshine and roses. Many people do it because it is easier to pile on the layers of protection, rather than deal with whatever is keeping them in their safe zones.

Your mental and physical health suffer under the umbrella of your "heroes cape." You don't want to burden anyone with what you are experiencing. You don't want others to know why you are putting on a mask, when behind it you are hurting. I am not going to pretend to know what has happened to you, or anyone else who is reading this book. It is not my place to know what you are going through. I can share what has been shared with me, but it may not even come close to what you are feeling. I can also be sympathetic and offer you a safe place, where you can lower your elephant-sized suitcase. I may even help you by getting rid of some of your baggage. At the end of a very long day, you are the one who has the authority and power to make the changes that will benefit you.

Health: Weighed Down Under the Baggage

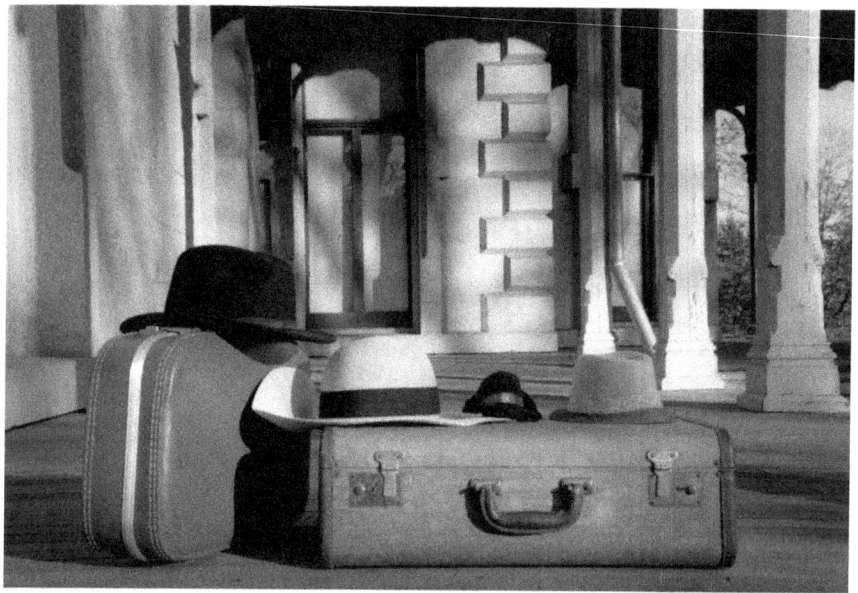

STOP! I would like you to hang on for a minute before you stand up, reach for your elephant-sized luggage, and storm off. I promised that I would not force anyone to do anything that they were not comfortable with. And I will keep my promise, on the condition that you listen to what I have to say. I know that you have well-meaning family and friends who want what is best for you. Let's take a moment to appreciate your special group of people who will do anything to help you, whether it be with advice or recommendations. I know that all you want is to scream and let everyone know that you don't want their help. This is where I start sliding in a few gentle reminders for anyone who hasn't been through a traumatic or hurtful event in their lives. I would like to share a few tips with well-meaning family and friends here:

- Take a step back.

- Don't smother the person you are 'helping.'

- Don't force your opinions on anyone.

- Don't dismiss the person.

- Don't force the person to speak about what is going on.

- Help by listening without telling them what to do and offering advice.

Let's take a look at what carrying the elephant-sized suitcase can do for your health. Remember that the weight being lugged around, like any physical weight, will present you with health concerns. Everyone knows what it is like to pick up a couple of extra pounds around the waist, hips, and thighs. We can lay the blame on midnight snack attacks in the pantry or refrigerator, or late-night visits to the gas station for that super-sized bar of Hershey chocolate, a bag of Nerd Clusters, or a packet of *Flamin' Hot Cheetos*. We are well acquainted with the 'damage' that eating junk food or overindulging does to our bodies.

No one wants to acknowledge the damage that is caused by shoving their feelings into a bottle. The phrase, "out of sight," comes to mind as you plaster some more anger, hatred, pain, or sadness into your bottle. I want to give you a look at what happens when you, or someone you care about, is unable or unwilling to let go. Your health and well-being is important to your loved ones. This is not a scare tactic, nor is it a ploy to get you to forgive someone—that is something that will come when you, and only you, are ready to take the next steps. Many people have fallen prey to carrying around more layers of unforgiveness than is necessary.

Cortisol: The Stress Regulator

I am in awe at what the human body goes through. We don't give our bodies the care and consideration they require. Have you ever thanked your body for giving you protection against the elements of nature? Have you ever considered why you would go from sobbing to laughing in minutes? Did you know that your body produces a steroid hormone known as cortisol? Let me tell you what cortisol means for you, me, and every person roaming around on this earth.

Cortisol is a steroid hormone that is produced by the adrenal glands. The adrenal glands are located on top of your kidneys, and are known as the endocrine glands. When cortisol is produced, it is released into the bloodstream and dispersed to various parts of the body. Cortisol is important to our bodies, because it helps to regulate any stress we may experience. It also helps the metabolism by controlling where the fats, proteins, and carbohydrates are transferred to in our bodies. Cortisol plays an important role in regulating blood pressure and blood sugar levels, and ensuring that our bodies get enough sleep.

Your kidneys are unable to keep up with the supply and demand that your body needs to regulate. Stress levels, holding onto unnecessary baggage, or adding debilitating emotions will affect your cortisol. You may argue that you are not experiencing any type of health issues, or that you are as fit as a fiddle. Most people refuse to accept that they are harboring any type of residual effects of whatever grudges or bitterness they are holding onto. It is a natural response for anyone who is, and has been, hiding in that jungle. You won't know what is hiding between the branches of the jungle if you don't acknowledge how you are really—honestly—feeling. Follow me as we trudge through parts of the jungle you don't want to see. You can hide behind me, because you know you can trust that I will protect you (Cleveland Clinic, 2021).

Memory

Do you remember being a student at school or university? Do you remember how you felt during the weeks or days leading up to the finals? You spent hours studying, maybe even memorizing, everything. The day of your exam arrives, you sit down to take your test, and you hit a blank. You have done nothing but study for weeks, and in the blink of an eye, you forget everything you have learned. You put so much pressure on yourself that your mind stops working. You may repeat a mantra or start breathing to calm your pounding heart. Your mind slowly starts waking up from its momentary panic, and you can take your exam.

It is not as easy for people who hold onto, and pile on, the layers of traumatic experiences. I spoke to someone who spent two weeks looking for a breadboard. They turned their kitchen upside down looking for this board. Two weeks and a couple of days later, they were standing at the kitchen basin and looked at the kitchen from a different angle. The kitchen was the cleanest and most organized than it had ever been—but wait, what did they spot? That's right, the breadboard was in a place that they had cleaned, scrubbed, and repacked multiple times during two weeks. This same person misplaced their sugar bowl. They searched high and low, and they were convinced that the sugar bowl had moved on to another family. It was becoming embarrassing to pass around a mug with sugar for their guests. After what seemed like forever, they found the sugar bowl in a place they had been in and out of multiple times during the day—the refrigerator. Today, this person is a work in progress and has finally started sorting through their luggage. They are far from where they need to be, but any progress is excellent for their health and well-being.

Hiding Behind the Habit-Forming Wall

It is easier to hide behind the habit-forming wall that offers protection, regardless of the negative effects of the habits. Stress and holding onto baggage wreak havoc on our cortisol levels. I have found that people are quick to point a crooked finger of criticism, judgment, and condemnation at those who do things that are frowned upon. The 'transgressions' I am referring to are people who may be smokers, drinkers, drug addicts, have eating disorders (overeating or starving themselves), or are self-mutilators. This list of 'transgressions' is a short list of what people go through. The most common reasons for people to adopt these habits is because of fear, anger, stress, or anxiety based on whatever traumatic experiences they have faced. We have those well-meaning individuals who will aggressively argue that people are stronger than what they believe, and they are looking for reasons to hide behind the safety of the habit-forming walls. Does any of what I have mentioned sound familiar to you? I'm pretty sure we are on the same page, because everyone has been there at some point during their lifetime.

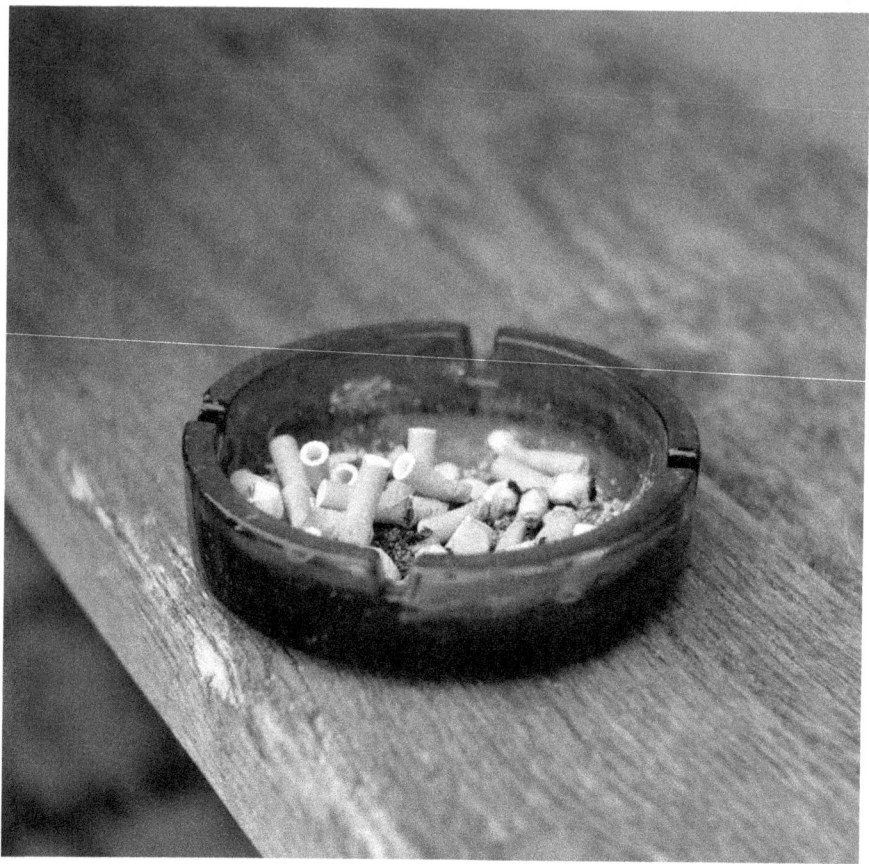

I interviewed someone who was more than happy to share their stories with me. This story is by no means meant to intimidate anyone. They are testimonials of this person I spoke with, who I found to be honest, truthful, and exuded compassion for everyone. In late 2000, they started smoking. When asked why they started smoking, they would not hesitate to lay all the blame on their children. They would say that the children and their friends were driving them up the wall, and they needed the escape. As you are aware, smoking is frowned upon across the board. The more this person was told what smoking was doing to them, the more they smoked. When the world became unhinged during a certain global pandemic, and everyone was forced to stay at home, they tried to stop smoking. It was hard.

Things took a turn when they joined an online church. They tried, without success, to stop smoking every other week. Sadly, the cease-fire would last a couple of days, at most. Stop-and-start smoking became a joke to this person's circle of friends. Wanting to get away from the butt of the jokes, they spent more time listening to podcasts and reconnecting with their faith. The weeks leading up to August 17th, 2021, made this person think about what it was that prevented them from getting rid of their smelly habit. On August 15th, the Pastor read a testimonial from someone whose story seemed to replicate theirs. They spoke about how they let go of damaged baggage, and the moment they did, things started changing.

This person knew what their damaged baggage was, and started to unpack it. Tuesday, August 17th, arrived without any fanfare. This person woke up, walked to the kitchen, lit up a cigarette, and was instantly repulsed by the smell coming from between their fingers. An hour later, they tried again, and this time they felt sick because the taste in their mouth was disgusting. That was the sign they had been waiting for. They gathered up their cigarettes, ashtray, and lighter, and tossed them in the trash. Almost nine months later, they hadn't been tempted to smoke again, because they realized that smoking was a crutch that was holding them back. This person doesn't take credit for giving up their smoking habit, instead they give all the credit to God. They added that they could never tell someone else what they should be doing with their lives, because everyone has to make a decision without being forced to. It was a process that they needed to go through, and do what was right for them at the right time.

Chapter 2:

How to Get Through the Pain, Heartache, and Anger Associated With Trauma

Welcome to the next leg of our journey together. I would like to start this chapter by inserting a trigger warning for everyone who is, and has been, affected by trauma. This chapter is dedicated to the brave people who are survivors of physical, mental, or emotional abuse. Trauma can be likened to a parasitic infection that may or may not leave you with long-lasting side effects. No one can hurt you or intimidate you while you are on this journey with me. This book is your safe space where you can put down your elephant-sized suitcase and take a well-deserved breather.

Forgiving someone is not as easy as one may believe it to be. My mythical tropical island fund jar would be overflowing with all the suggestions of how I should forgive people for what they have done to me. Some may find it easier than others to push that forgiveness button. Others may be trying to make sense of what happened, and need time to process what happened. There is more to trauma than being physically, mentally, or emotionally abused. Trauma has no boundaries, and it will latch on to anyone who is vulnerable. Some would refer to the vulnerable as pushovers, and others may say that they are kind and compassionate. The list of traumatic experiences is never-ending, and includes the following:

- a spouse having an affair
- fraudulent activity on your bank account

- a loved one stealing from you to feed a habit

- physical, mental, and emotional abuse from close friends or family

- sexual abuse or molestation by family or friends

- sexual abuse or assault by trusted members of the community or strangers

- aggravated robbery

- the murder of a friend, family member, or a member of the community

- the diagnosis of a life-threatening illness

This list doesn't come close to all the different types of traumas people experience. I want people to know that they don't have to hide in shame from the trauma that they have been exposed to or endured. You have a right, and the choice, to use your voice to help others by sharing your experience. I have previously mentioned that you are stronger than you give yourself credit for. I recently found a YouTube video of an incident that happened in 2018. The video is titled: *"Mom Comes Face-To-Face With Her Son's Killer In Court."* I don't know what I was expecting when I clicked on the video, but I will admit that I was pleasantly surprised by the outcome.

The lady's son was murdered by a teenager, who left him to die in the gutter. The mom embraces her son's murderer and tells him that she forgives him. She approaches each of his family members and either shakes their hands, gives them hugs, or does both. When the lady gets to the teenager's mother, I had tears streaming down my face, because the interaction between both mothers showed the pain each was suffering. On the one hand, we have a mother who was mourning the death of her son—and on the other hand, we have a mother who was mourning her son for a crime he had committed. The mother of the murdered son says that there is no point in seeking revenge. She continues by saying that revenge doesn't solve anything. The brave mother says that she can't hate the teenager, because hate doesn't feature in her religion.

I decided to share this story at the beginning of this chapter, because I wanted to show you how a grieving mother can forgive someone for violently taking her son away. She forgave the teenager, but neither of them will ever be able to forget what had happened. The teenager has to live with what he has done for the rest of his life, and there is nothing worse than being saddled with a guilty conscience. Yes, the teenager can forgive himself for what he had done, but the memory of what happened will be with him forever. The whole scenario could have turned out differently, and the mother of the innocent victim could have spewed hatred and said how much she hoped he suffered a fate worse than her son's.

Do What Is Right for You, and Not for Anyone Else

I didn't share the mother's story to bully, intimidate, or force you into a corner. I would never do that to anyone. You don't have to be like the mother and forgive the person who hurt you. You are allowed to be angry at the person, or people, who hurt you. You may have murderous thoughts about those who hurt you. You are allowed to experience all the feelings associated with whatever happened to you. I may not be a medical professional, but I am a survivor of traumatic experiences and events in my own lifetime. I may or may not have walked around like an atomic bomb. I know what it feels like to carry around an elephant-sized suitcase that is filled with negative, hateful, angry, and sad feelings. That is one of the reasons why I decided to write this book—I wanted to show people that they don't have to do anything until they are ready. The victim is the most important person in this book. The victim doesn't have to be someone who was physically, mentally, or emotionally abused. The victim can be anyone who has been hurt because of someone disrespecting or dismissing them, being lied to, or being led around in circles with no regard for other's feelings.

Identifying Physical and Emotional Symptoms of Traumatic Stress

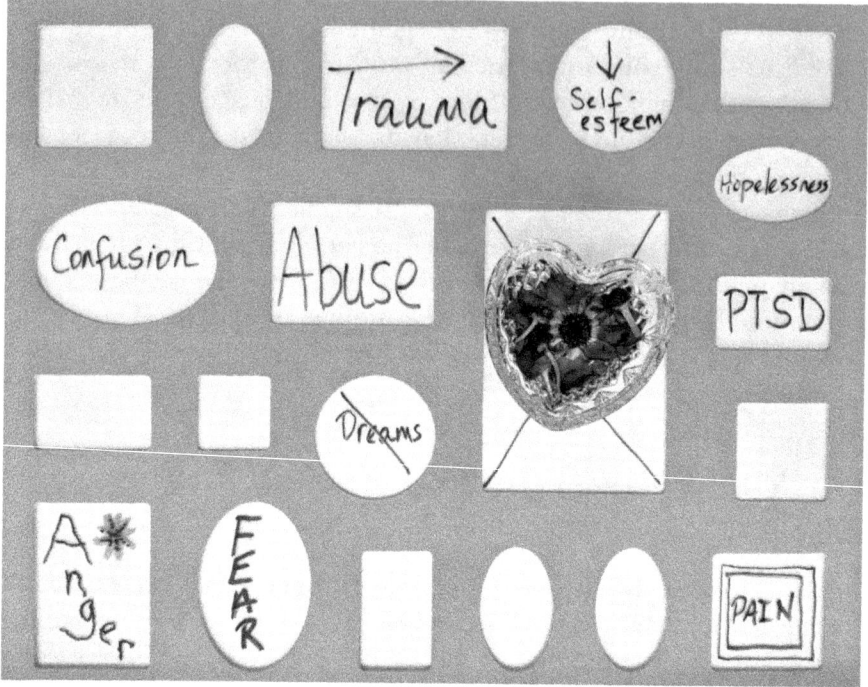

You, and only you, have the power to do what is right for your circumstances. You get to lay down the ground rules, because this is your journey. You can add or remove whomever and whatever you decide does not respect what you represent. Come a little closer and pay very close attention to what I have to say; this is not about your family, friends, acquaintances, or strangers—this is about *YOU!* Someone recently told me that you don't have to give anyone a reason when you choose to stand up for yourself. You don't have to validate the reasons for doing what you do. You have to do what is right for you. I will admit that I am one of those who is taken advantage of quite frequently. I don't do or say anything until I reach the stage where my patience, generosity, and understanding nature has reached its limits. Most people don't understand the trauma involved when standing up for oneself. I have met people who visibly pale when faced with the idea of standing up for themselves. No one knows the amount of pressure the victims stack on their shoulders because they want to avoid confrontations.

I would like to show you some of the effects and symptoms of what physical and emotional stress may add to your life. Please remember that the trigger warning I issued at the beginning of this chapter is still in effect. I believe that it is time to show others what traumatized victims may be lugging around on their shoulders. You may want to leave your book open on the following couple of pages, so that someone else can get a glimpse of what you are reading about. You may not be ready or want to talk about your feelings, but it is a good stepping stone to alert people as to what you are looking at. Who knows, they might even come forward and make amends, or start a conversation that will be helpful to you. Please note that I am not a medical professional, but I am someone who has been through the mill. The remainder of this chapter will be based on medically-backed information from medical professionals who practice, and are trained in, the fields of post-traumatic stress disorder (PTSD) and traumatic stress cases.

Anxiety

Anxiety is a physical and emotional reaction to carrying around unnecessary stress. I like using the analogy of a can of soda that has been shaken around. The can has space for a certain amount of fluid before adding the carbonation and being sealed. When the can is opened, you can hear the 'pop' and the hissing of the bubbles. We all know what happens when the can is agitated by shaking, tossing it to someone, leaving it in a heated car, or even putting it in the freezer. The moment you pop the tab on the can, you have to take cover or you run the risk of being a victim of the angry soda spraying all over. If you happen to (accidentally or on purpose) put the can of soda in the freezer, you are going to need a whole lot of cleaning materials—because you will be facing a disaster of epic proportions.

People who suffer from anxiety attacks don't like talking about it, because they are afraid of people judging them. It is very important to understand that no two people will have the same experiences. I don't like drawing attention to myself, and I certainly do not want to be placed under a microscope. I can normally sense when an attack is imminent, and eight out of ten times, I can distract myself enough to avoid one. Not everyone is as lucky as I am, though. I realize that I am making this sound like a walk through the forest, but it took many years for me to learn various techniques. I went from having three attacks a week to approximately one attack every three months. Some days are easier than others, but for someone who is a victim of different types of stressful situations, it is a work in progress—constantly working on new techniques.

The following list of symptoms may all be linked together under the anxiety umbrella, or they may be standalone symptoms of stress. Since I do not have a medical degree, what I am sharing is my personal experience. Please consult your general practitioner or medical professional for a diagnosis.

- The feeling that your heart wants to escape out of your chest.

- Your mind is constantly thinking about the worst-case scenario which can prevent you from sleeping, make you paranoid, or cause confusion.

- Struggling to catch your breath or breathe rapidly.

- Struggling with insomnia, experiencing nightmares, or wanting to sleep all day.

- Hiding behind your habit-forming wall, as discussed in Chapter 1.

Emotional Grab Bag

I know that "grab bag" does not embody any medical term in any of the textbooks, but I do believe that emotions represent a lucky packet. You never know which emotion will surface at whatever time of the day or night, or what emotion will rear its delightfully (un)pleasant head. I can't help but mention the hectic world we live in, and the expectations everyone has to live up to. Everyone has forgotten how to hit the pause button on the merry-go-round that we so lovingly call life. One of my experiences with humankind is that people have lost the ability to have a decent conversation while looking at the person they are with. A decent conversation, in my eyes, is putting your mobile phone on silent, placing it in your bag, and looking at the person sitting across from you. The human interaction connection has been damaged. I believe that this is one of the many reasons why people act surprised when they learn that their family members, or friends, are experiencing PTSD or traumatic stress. I'm not telling anyone what to do, but I am sharing my beliefs from what I have observed.

Let's take a look in the grab bag of emotional traumatic stress symptoms to see what may or may not resonate with what you are feeling:

- shame
- guilt
- sadness
- grief
- fear
- anger
- shock
- a feeling of helplessness
- relief

Recovering From Trauma May Be Easier Than You Think

This is an excellent introduction to the rest of the book, and what you can expect going forward. I will not be browbeating you, and I will not use any type of force. You are in control of the remote, and you can press pause at any point during this journey we call recovery. I have introduced you to the many different symptoms that you could be struggling with, which you didn't know about. You are very aware that this book is about you making peace with painful memories, which include—but are not limited to—the list I mentioned at the beginning of this chapter. I have shared my struggles with anxiety. I will also be sharing some of my tried and tested coping tools throughout the rest of this book.

The medical professionals have shared their expertise on how to deal with traumatic stress situations. The information I will be sharing mimics most of what I have, and will, be dropping in upcoming chapters. It is important to remember that what will work for me may not work for you—and what works for Annie at the local Dunkin' outlet won't work for someone who had a motor vehicle accident. Whatever you are struggling with is unique to you, and should not be dismissed by yourself or anyone else.

I spoke to a lady who wanted to share her story with others. Her story may not be all that unique, because it is something everyone is aware of, and has been part of in some way or another. We all know that new moms don't have it all that easy. The friends who don't have children are not available at the drop of a hat—and to be fair, you don't want to cart your child/ren around while your child/ren entertain themselves. The best solution is to find other mom friends.

The lady was deathly afraid of stepping out of her comfort zone and looking for people who have children who are close in age to her own child. Stepping out of one's comfort zone is very traumatic and very brave. The lady met a mom who introduced her to other moms, and that was the beginning of a brand-new group of friends… A year goes by, and the lady notices that the dynamics of this mom group have radically changed. She is no longer being invited to join the other moms, and her son is excluded from all activities. This goes on for a couple more months until she sees one of the newer members of the group, and is left in awe at the attitude of this person when she wanted to introduce herself. She was condescending, rude, and looked down at her as she told her—in front of the other moms—that she wasn't talking to her. Taken off guard, the lady started crying because she was in shock—as well as confused, because she didn't know what had happened for someone to treat her so poorly.

The lady told me that she was filled with all types of emotions. She kept asking herself and her husband what could be the reason for the expulsion from the group? She wanted to know if she wasn't cool enough to be part of the group? Had she unknowingly offended someone without realizing it? Was there something wrong with the type of clothes she wore? Had her child done something to the other children? She wanted to know what she or her child had done, so that she could rectify the situation.

It took weeks for her to understand that she didn't do anything wrong. After weeks of carrying around a range of emotions, she made peace with the situation and was actually relieved. The weight had been lifted from her shoulders. She didn't have to put on airs and graces, and pretend to be someone she was not. She shares, with a smile on her face, that she made a new group of 'real' mom friends; and the fake mom friends have built up quite a stellar reputation in their small town—not a very good one.

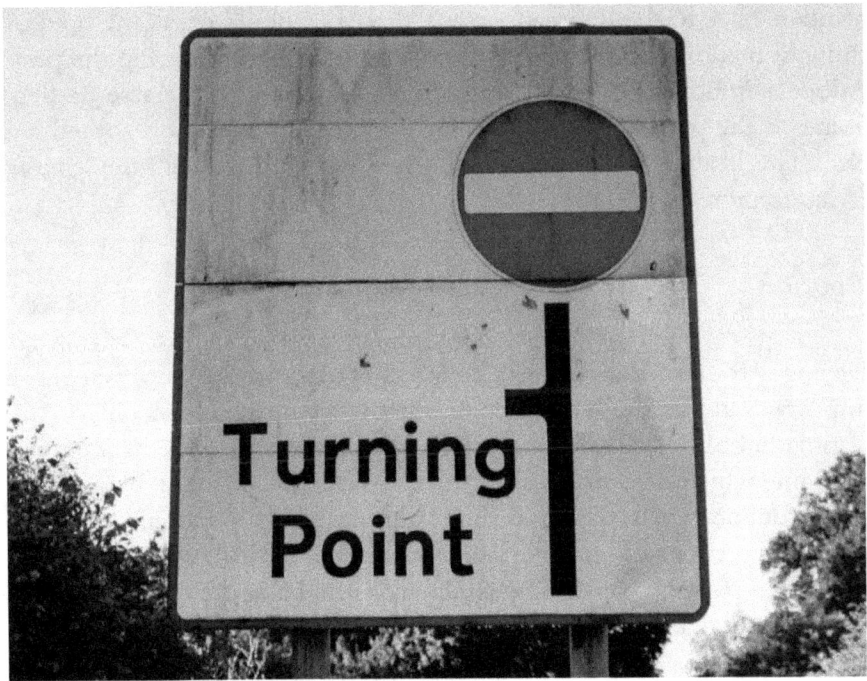

Small Steps in the Right Direction

You may be raising your eyes and wondering if there is a right direction. The answer depends on you. You have to ask yourself if you want to move past whatever is holding you hostage, or whether you are happy being in that invisible cage. I'm not a fortune teller, but I'm pretty certain you want to break free from whatever is holding you in its clutches. I need you to read and believe what I am telling you, and that is—you need to be kind to yourself. The best and most effective way for you to do that is to ease up on yourself. Loosen the reins on the guilt, anger, fear, or sadness you are dragging around with you. It is okay to let go. It is not a competition to see who can carry around the most physical or emotional baggage. Let's see what the medical experts have to say about dropping some of this baggage.

Reprogram Your Mind

This one may be asking a lot—but in the interest of your health and well-being, it is important. It is suggested that whenever your mind wanders back to the traumatic event, that you should break the train of thought by doing an activity. It is not healthy to keep reliving the past. Adopt a hobby such as cooking, baking, starting a vegetable garden, going to the gym, or anything that will help you focus on something else. The healing will begin when you stop spending all your energy trying to recreate the past.

Routine

Having a routine is an excellent idea in today's world, but even more important in the life of someone who is trying to come out of the trauma bubble. A routine will establish some much-needed stability in your life, which incorporates normalcy. We all know that a baby needs a set routine for feeding, sleeping, tummy time, or bathing. It helps them feel secure and, in some ways, provides a sense of security. Adults can take a page out of the day-to-day life of a baby; learn how to build a routine that offers safety, security, and peace that is necessary for healing.

Don't Make Hasty Decisions

I know, from experience, that you should not be making any major life changes when you are in the throes of your traumatic experience. I have spoken to many people who have told me about their regret at having sold their house because they couldn't imagine living it after the death of a partner or a child. The bottom line is that when you do things in haste, you don't think about the possible ramifications of what you could be doing to yourself or those involved in making these decisions. Remove yourself from the stressful situation, but don't think of doing anything in haste until you have reached the point where you can successfully separate your emotions from your surrounding reality (Smith, M. et al., 2021b).

Chapter 3:

Why You Should Cut Yourself

Some Slack

Welcome to the next stop on this island-hopping tour. I love virtual reality scenarios because I can go anywhere, be or do anything, and I don't have to worry about offending anyone. Virtual reality offers me a safe space where I don't have to be brave. No one, other than myself, can hurt me in my world of virtual reality. I can hit the pause button whenever I need to. Escaping into my virtual reality allows me to evaluate where I am in my life's journey. I get to let down my guard. I get to slouch my shoulders. In short, I get to take a break from everything that is weighing me down. I will be the first to openly admit that it is not easy to set down the elephant-sized suitcase.

The next stop on this island-hopping tour is going to be about everyone opening the luggage they have been dragging around. We are going to put on brave faces and take little steps outside of the virtual reality world that has been a protective zone for longer than anyone can remember. We are going to do something that may make you shudder in fear—and that is sorting through the items you have been carrying around with you. You are going to learn how to separate the items into piles by order of relevance. I know that each of the items you have stuffed into your elephant-sized suitcase plays an important role in your life. Always remember that you do have a choice in what happens in your life. Don't ever be afraid to stand up for what you believe in. Don't back down because you are being intimidated. Help is always just around the corner and will be there when you need it.

I'm not here to tell you what you should or shouldn't be doing with your life. However, I would like to show you the view from a survivor's point of view. Yes, this book is about forgiveness. No, I am not going to force you to forgive someone. I know that forgiving someone is very difficult. I can't speak for you or the situation you are going through, but I *can* be that annoying voice of reason. The voice that wants you to know that you do not have to carry around the burden of whatever is holding you hostage. I'm going to share my point of view with you, and you may disagree with me. I would like to implore you to see the world through the eyes of people who have gone through the depths of the jungles in which you currently find yourself entangled. I like to remind my readers to always have an open mind, and not act without seeing the view from the other side of the lens.

The Effects of Dealing With Pain

I touched on the damage of having higher cortisol levels and what it could mean for your overall health; but I never got around to exploring the long-term side effects of holding onto the weight that comes with the emotional baggage. You tell everyone that all is fine and dandy in your world. You plaster on the best fake smile pain can buy. You allow people to believe that nothing phases you. No one knows that your shining armor of bravery comes apart when you step into your virtual reality. The fake smile disintegrates. The elephant-sized suitcase explodes. You look around to find that everything you stuffed into your luggage is strewn around. You allow yourself to be vulnerable for a couple of hours as you prepare to repeat the process.

It is true that no one knows what you may be going through. It is true that each person finds themselves trapped in their invisible case. I know what it feels like to take all the pain that accompanies emotional baggage. I know all about the guilt that is stuffed into that elephant-sized suitcase we carry around on our shoulders. Guilt is like an infected wound that cannot heal without the proper medication. I find that I have to bite down on my teeth to stop myself from telling someone what their actions or words have done to me. These people have no trouble or shame in carrying on with their daily lives, while others hide away from what they have done. You may even find yourself screaming (silently, of course) that they are liars and don't have an inch of remorse. I believe that we know such people, and the scary part of it is—they may even be related to us by blood.

Compartmentalizing the Contents of the Emotional Baggage

I was chatting with my publisher, and they told me about someone they work with who is a 'chronic' hoarder. I laughed, because it was a term I had never heard before. They told me that the person—whom I will name Alex—stored everything in their mind. They collected every bit of information they could. Alex had compartments in their mind where everything would go. Former employers would regularly call them up to find out dates, "Can you remember what I did with this, that, or the other," or the directions they took to get somewhere. Another compartment was filled with memories of what Alex had experienced during their formative years. They could share every important and memorable event of their life, from before they were three years of age. Most people cannot even remember what they ate for breakfast.

Alex's mental compartments multiplied as the years went by. The compartments consisted of both good and bad memories. Alex was a very private person who didn't look for attention. They preferred to stay in the shadows. They are the type of person that everyone knows is there, and that they are always on hand to help others. This is what makes others take advantage of a good person. Everyone knows where they can find the broad shoulders, the caring heart, and the nonjudgmental ear. They didn't like to share what they were going through, but they were always willing to take on other people's troubles, and stuff them in their elephant-sized suitcases.

I needed to know why Alex would take on other people's burdens. The curiosity bug was working overtime—and when it starts tickling, you know you have to find out more. They were more than happy to share their story with me, and I did get permission to share their story. I asked many questions, especially about the compartments my publisher had spoken about. They told me that over the years, they had experienced a lot of bullying during their time in school at the hands of classmates, and even teachers. They suffered bullying at the hands of aunts, uncles, cousins, grandparents, and siblings. Alex said that even though they were hurt by what everyone was doing and saying, they just stored everything into compartments and stayed silent. They were aware of the physical effects of what compartmentalizing everything was doing to their lives. They did what we spoke about in the previous chapter, and found safety by building habit-forming walls. Alex developed an unhealthy relationship with food, which prompted the bullying to become even worse.

I learned a lot from Alex. Their story may seem familiar to yours, and it may even mimic what you are going through. You may want to stick around to see what we can learn from Alex. They also shared the lessons that helped them let go of one compartment at a time. They mentioned that the elephant-sized suitcase they carry around has gotten considerably lighter over the course of the last couple of years. This is a testimony that everything will play out as, and when it is, necessary. It is a process that cannot be rushed, and everyone needs to start lightening the load somewhere. You should have realistic goals, and not measure your progress against anyone else's. How can *YOU* implement the first steps of your healing process? Oh, I'm so happy that you asked! Please follow me as I show you how you can start lightening the load you are carrying around.

How to Limit Excess Luggage

Everyone has packed for an overnight sleepover, a business trip, or a vacation at some point in their lives. Almost everyone I know detests packing, because they either pack too much or too little. I have friends who make extensive lists that tell everyone what they will be wearing on which day, what their accessories are going to be, and what socks and shoes they will need. The next list is for the toiletry bag, which is for the essential hygiene products such as toothbrushes, toothpaste, facecloths, and whatever else is needed. The essentials such as shampoo, conditioner, facial products, makeup, and a first aid kit is Mom's responsibility. This is a very well-organized system that many will follow, but also not get it 100% correct. No shame Mom, you are human, and it is slightly less than impossible to ensure that you've packed everything. These are also the group of people who weigh their luggage to ensure that they stick within the parameters of the weight limits if they are traveling by air.

Another type of person is the one who packs everything in the house, including the dishwasher, because what if their vacation rental doesn't have one—only joking (almost). You get the idea, though. The suitcases are bulging, and it takes at least two adults to secure the latches. Heaven forbid that the suitcase explodes mid-journey. You suddenly realize that you have packed some tattered and soiled laundry from the washing basket. Your mind goes into overdrive, because all the "what-ifs" are threatening to jump out of the suitcase to flaunt your laundry in front of everyone. Do you want to be that person who lives in fear? Of course, you don't. I want to show you what type of life you can expect for yourself if you were to start sorting through and getting rid of tattered and soiled laundry.

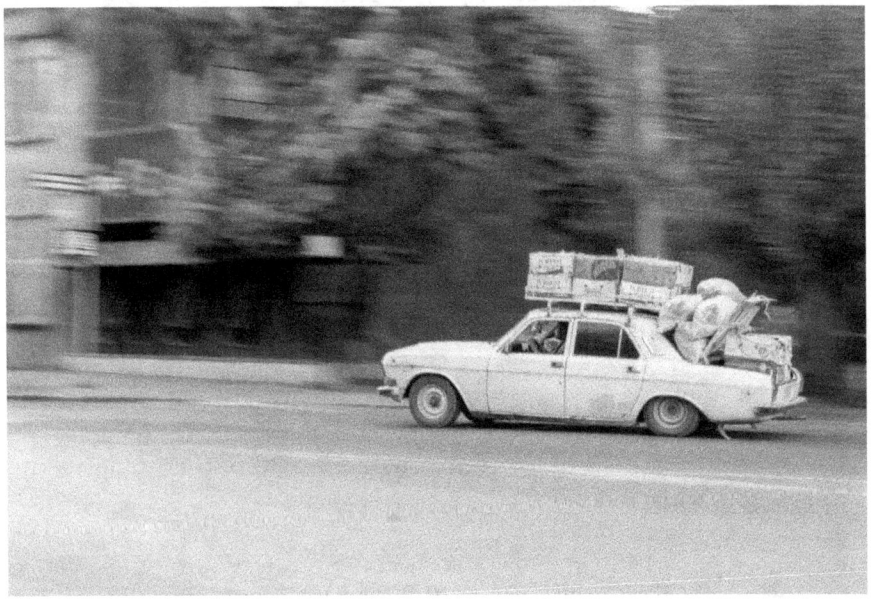

Each piece of laundry you remove from your elephant-sized suitcase could potentially be beneficial to your physical and mental health. You may want to bring a notebook and pen for the next part. I'm one of those who loves making lists when it comes to my life, and what's going on in it. Make a list, go over it a couple of times, and see what speaks to you. See where you can trim some of the toxicity in your life. I am not going to put you in harm's way, either. I will show you some techniques that you can use, if you wish, to forgive those who hurt you without ever seeing them or speaking to them. You don't owe anyone anything, but you owe yourself everything. I am not going to *kumbaya* you into doing something that you aren't ready for, either. I was going to insert my annoying gentle reminder, but I think it is safe to assume that you know that I have your back.

Recognition

This is where you get to step into your mind and take a look around. You need to find and identify at least one of the incidents where you were hurt. Write down everything you can remember from that time. Even the smallest detail will help you. Ask yourself questions as you rummage through your mind.

- Who stole the light out of my eyes?

- Who replaced the light with fear, sadness, or anger?

- Who was it that hurt me to the point where I am afraid to be myself?

- Was I intentionally hurt or was I just being overly sensitive?

- Did someone say something to hurt my feelings?

- Did I take a comment out of context without listening to the whole story?

Ask yourself whatever questions you need to, so that you can pinpoint why you are feeling the way you are. You and whoever hurt you, whether intentionally or unintentionally, will know the truth. I did say that you didn't have to face anyone you didn't want to. Take a deep breath and calm down. This section of the book needs you to recognize the trigger, so that healing can begin. What you ultimately want to achieve is a lighter load, and regain the sparkle in your eyes. When you achieve the goal of a lighter load, you will start seeing the space around you a little clearer because you are standing a little taller. Please remember that this is a book, and it is not going to hurt you. Everything you find from the very first page, right up to the image reference list at the end of the book is free of judgment, bullying, and condemnation. You will find compassion, understanding, and as much support as you need.

Addressing Whoever Hurt You

Take a couple of deep breaths, please. This section is not what you think it is. I know this may be painful, but I want you to find an item in your home that you can speak to. It can be anything you choose. Set the item up so that you are sitting across from it, and tell this item how you are feeling. This is your stage, and you can say or do whatever you want. Be angry, scream, or cry. Unscrew the bottle of soda you have been carrying around in your suitcase. Let it spray everywhere. Venting is one of the best methods of healing, because you don't have anyone interrupting you.

The next step on the path of healing is one that I love. I have heard of many people using this method, which has helped them to move on from the chains that were choking them. I would recommend the old-fashioned way of writing, which is with a pen and paper, but you can use any of your devices. Write a letter to whoever hurt you. Don't hold back in your letter to them. It is important for you to let out everything that you have been holding in. Tell them how you feel. You do whatever you need to do. The choices you have are pretty simple. You can send the letter to the person via the postal service, email, or have someone hand-deliver it. Instead of having anyone read what you have written, you could also burn the letter as part of a cleansing ritual. I will share more about rituals and practices in Chapter 7—don't worry, there will be no voodoo and no harming of individuals.

What Is So Wonderful About Living in the Past?

I will be the first to admit that the past needs to stay where it is. Truth be told, you can't travel back in time to change whatever has happened. I am always telling people you can't unring a bell. You can, however, shape the future to make it a better place. Yes, you were hurt. No one knows what you have been through. Alex said something that made sense to me at the time. They said that they had made a promise not to be angry with a family member. The family member has been spreading stories about the siblings, and played one up against the other. Alex's mother passed away, and they were angry. They promised that they wouldn't hold a grudge against the person who continues to spread malicious lies. Alex held onto the grudge, even though they loved the person dearly, for seven very long years. When that pandemic hit the shores all across the globe, Alex knew that they had to implement the, *forgive them, for they do not know what they are doing...* verse from the New International Version of Luke 23:34. Alex said goodbye to their loved one and whispered in their ear that they forgive them, because they knew that they would never see their loved one alive again. Their loved one passed away with a smile on their face six months later. They were finally free from the past because, while everyone else was continuing the feud, Alex had taken the all-important step to forgive. Alex said that the morning they received the message of the passing, they felt as if a boulder had been removed from their shoulder.

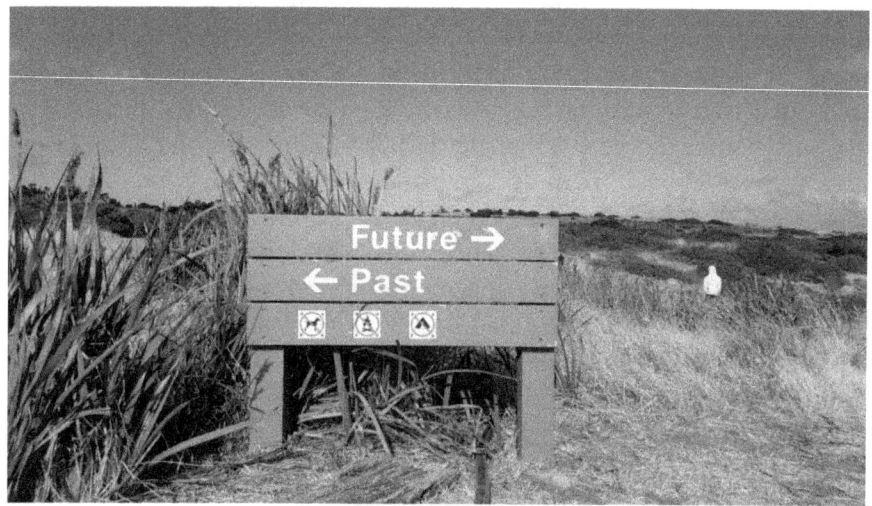

Chapter 4:

Learning How to Forgive

This may be one of the most intimidating islands on this journey. I know that you are shaking with fear as you prepare to take your first step onto the island. This is the island experience you may have been hoping to avoid, and rightfully so. I want to reassure you, as I have been doing since you embarked on this journey, that no one can or will hurt you here. Find a spot where you can set down your jumbo-sized suitcase. And yes, your suitcase is getting lighter because you have chosen to lighten the load. You are beginning to feel at ease, knowing that you are the victim, and understanding that you can make the necessary changes. I want you to disembark from this cruise carrying a purse. I want to prepare you for what to expect going forward, so that you don't feel ambushed. Be sure to stick around for more details relating to this bit of information I have shared. Right now, I am only doing what any caring person would do, and that is preparing you for the future.

Right, your suitcase has been safely stored, you have had a moment to stretch, and have picked a flower from the vines of courage. You get to decide on your position as we trek through this jungle. You may, as you know, hide behind me whenever you are feeling anxious or afraid. You will begin to notice that the jungle is not as dense as it was when you first stepped onto the island. Together we are going to learn about a very important self-healing technique that will be beneficial to you, me, and everyone else who follows along on this journey. This is one of those techniques you either want to test out, or completely dismiss as nonsense. You know that you have choices, and no one can force you, or put pressure on you to choose. You may know by now that I like to share tiny nuggets of advice or secrets. The seed I want to plant in your mind is that this chapter does not require you to sign a contract holding you accountable for anything, nor does it require a subscription. You can go join us along this journey, learn some techniques you don't know, or find fault with all the suggestions I have to offer. As I said, you have choices, and it is up to you how you want to proceed going forward.

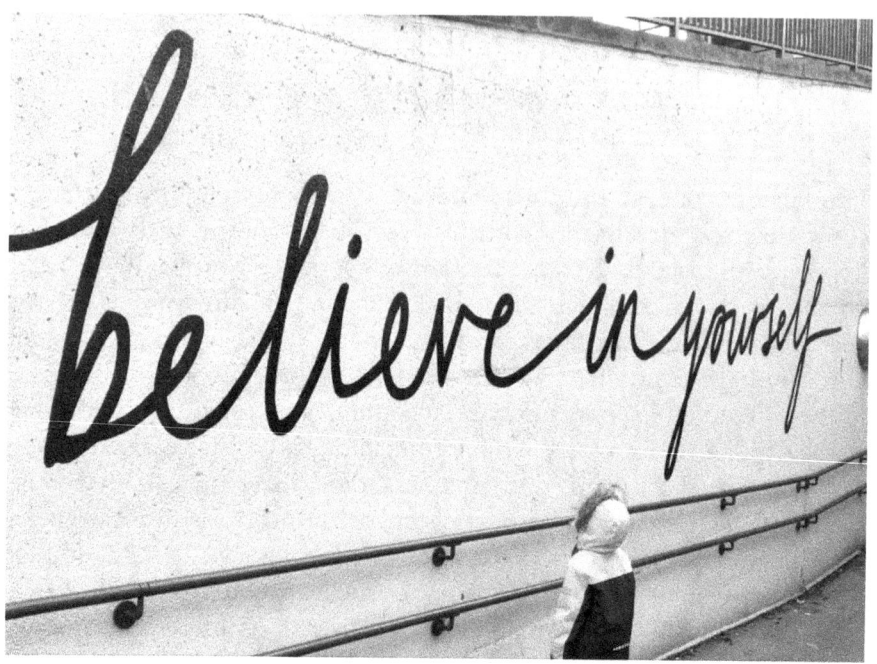

The Ins and Outs: Understanding and Benefits of Forgiveness

How can anyone be expected to forgive someone or something if they don't know what it means? You were taught how to say sorry from a very young age, without really understanding why you are saying it. You start growing and developing feelings in situations where sorry and, "please forgive me," is used a lot. Your bestie decides that they don't want to be friends anymore, and moves on to a new group. The new group laughs and jeers whenever you are nearby, and it makes you uncomfortable. It is not long before you are excluded from activities because of whatever gossip the new group spreads about you. Confusion, betrayal, and hurt enter the emotional feeling stage. You feel betrayed, because someone you were close with since kindergarten has dumped you for a group of not-so-nice friends. You are confused because you cannot understand why you are being made fun of. You are hurt because you don't know why they are picking on you when they don't know anything about you. Your former bestie sees that you avoid eye contact, and takes note of your slouched posture as you walk past them. Their conscience kicks in, they approach you, and ask you to, "please forgive me." What are you going to do? That is why I am writing this book.

I'm not here to give you information based on my beliefs. I do a lot of research about the topics I write about. Many may agree with me that information on websites, articles, or even videos has a way of losing its meaning because everything is so technical. I know many people who avoid reading certain topics because they don't enjoy reading textbook-style contexts. Some may say that it is pure laziness, and that people want everything to be simplified to avoid learning. Others may say that simplifying the subject they are learning about is beneficial to enriching their thought process, and understanding. I happen to throw my weight behind the second observation. It has nothing to do about being lazy, or not wanting to understand the topic of discussion. It has everything to do with helping people understand that they have options and choices. Simplifying content is not spoon-feeding anyone, it is about breaking down the textbook content—which some may say is boring—and giving it some body.

Understanding Forgiveness

My go-to resource for any definitions is the Merriam-Webster online dictionary. I consider us to be best friends (even though they don't know who I am), because I am always using them to help me express myself. The definition of forgiveness that I got from Merriam-Webster was pretty simple with its description; which was defined as putting an end to any of the negative emotional connotations against someone, or a circumstance where you were offended, hurt, or suffered any emotional damage from a situation. It's also used in the financial world wherein the debt will be written off by the lender of a monetary loan, or an agreement has been entered into by a friend to repay a loan and instead you decide to gift it (Merriam-Webster, n.d.).

I found an article that was written by the Mayo Clinic Staff titled: *Forgiveness: Letting go of grudges and bitterness*. I know that we are still entertaining the idea of introducing and applying forgiveness to our lives. This is where I will defend those who are hesitant about the idea of forgiveness, because this is not an easy topic. The reason why I have chosen this article is that one of the subheadings in the article actually asks: "What is forgiveness?" I thought that it was a good idea to share with you what the medical world has to say about forgiveness.

The Mayo Clinic Staff article says that the act of forgiving someone will have different meanings for different people or situations. The general understanding of forgiveness is that you have the choice to let go of the negative emotional connotations, such as feelings of wanting to get even, hatred, or fear. The article continues to remind readers that memories are not as easy to let go of, but forgiving someone for the acts done against you will help with your healing. I know that it is not easy to let go of whatever is holding you hostage, because you may believe that keeping that memory alive and active is your protection. You, and only you, can decide what it is that you want in this life (Mayo Clinic Staff, 2020).

- Do you want to continue living in fear?

- Do you want to go through a life that is fueled by hatred?

- Will revenge get back what was taken from you?

Think about the Mom I spoke about in Chapter 3. She had two choices. For her, it was a no-brainer. She could have stood in front of the teenager, pounded on his chest, clawed and slapped his face, or even spat at him while hurling profanities at him. She could have been screaming at his mother who was experiencing pain for what her child had done to someone else. Instead, the mother who lost the most precious gift in her life, chose to forgive because nothing will bring her son back. Revenge is not going to hurt someone else; it is only going to prevent you from enjoying your life today. Remember that you can't go back to yesterday, because there is nothing that you can do to change it. You can think about tomorrow, but don't spend too much time there because tomorrow will only happen tomorrow. Live today, and choose to make today your priority.

Benefits of Forgiveness

Everything we do in life comes with choices—or as some would say, rules. I think that we could divide the population into three categories: rule makers, rule followers, and rule breakers. I have to chuckle at the categories, because they represent the stages of our lives. Growing up, you have your parents and everyone older than you making the rules. The next stage of your life involves following the rules, until you are old enough to start breaking them. The next stage is about undoing everything you learned in stage one. Reality eventually catches up, and many revert back to stage two. Stages one, two, and three are on loop for the remainder of your life, because they are an integral part of your life. It all boils down to making choices that are beneficial to your current life.

I have touched on and hinted at the benefits of lightening the load you are carrying around on your shoulders. The article from the staff writers of the Mayo Clinic I mentioned in the previous section offers a list of why you should forgive someone. I know you are not ready to empty your jumbo-sized suitcase in one sitting, and I'm going to go out on a limb here, and say that no one else expects you to do it. Letting go is a traumatic experience, and it is not as easy as people believe it to be. I do get hurt and mildly angry when people tell me to forget about this, that, or the other, and, "just move on from," whatever is weighing me down. I can't begin to imagine how people who are physically, sexually, or emotionally traumatized must be feeling. I recently heard a young dad interacting with his five- or six-year-old son in the store. The son was having a 'moment' in the snack aisle, because he wanted something. The young dad crouched down to his son's level and recited part of a quote by Gloria Tesch, which I had heard many times before; *There is a time and place for everything, you just have to wait for the right moment.*

I thought that the quote was appropriate, and the son seemed to understand what his dad was saying. The little boy wiped away his tears, reached for his dad's hand, looked up at him, and gave him a big smile. That dad was definitely a rule maker, rule follower, and rule breaker, and he was teaching his son the same principles. The moral of my eyewitness experience is that, "there is a time and place for everything, you just have to wait for the right moment," and I believe that the right moment will be whenever you are comfortable. Here is a list, as shared by multiple medical professionals, of the benefits of forgiveness. For quick reference, write them down in your notebook, or you can bookmark this page (Mayo Clinic Staff, 2020):

- Anxiety and stress levels will become manageable.
- Your blood pressure will normalize.
- You are less likely to struggle with severe depression.
- Overall, your physical and mental health will improve.
- You will feel more confident.
- Your relationships with family and friends will improve.

The Blueprints for Your Healing Process

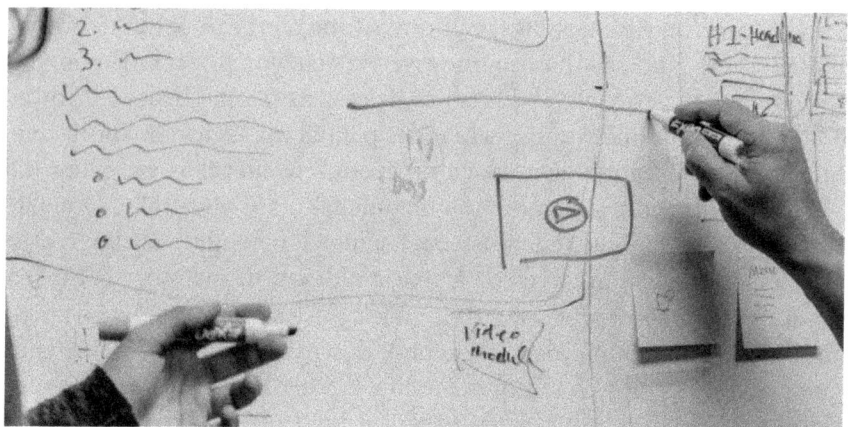

These blueprints are custom-made for your convenience, and tailor-made to suit your circumstances. Tweak them any way you want. Use the knowledge you are still to gain, add whatever you found helpful in previous chapters, or work on anything you feel I may have missed. The base of your blueprints will be positivity. That is the most important part of the blueprints, and it is not negotiable. You are the architect, and this is your journey. Your healing process will be determined by how you lighten the load that you carry around in your suitcase. It is your process to work through, with the advice or guidance explained in a simplified manner.

Remember that drawing up your blueprints will not cost you a dime. I'm sure that we are all very aware of the costs involved in hiring an architect. You will not have to sell a kidney, a sliver of your liver, or any other part of your body to work on these blueprints. All that you are going to learn during this process is that you need to have an open mind, and be positive. These two ticket items are the glue that is going to help prepare your mind, body, and soul for a gloriously peaceful future. Before we can proceed, I would just like to say that one of the items on your blueprints has been mentioned in this chapter—and that was to know and understand what forgiveness is, including the benefits. The second item on your blueprints has previously been mentioned at the beginning of Chapter 3, about the empathy of a mother whose son was violently taken from her life and this world.

Preparation

This step is going to cause your anxiety to go into overdrive. The thought of doing something where you had experienced intimidation can trigger emotions you have never experienced. Take yourself and the offender out of the equation, and look at your surroundings. Take a look around at the people you see in the store, at the library, at church, or in the parking area. Do something that will put a smile on someone's face. Carry a couple of mini candy bars in your bag and give them to someone who you think would need them. Give a neighbor a bunch of freshly picked flowers or freshly harvested vegetables from your garden. Smile at someone. You are spreading positivity, as well as building up your confidence.

Identifying the Pain

You are going to have to scratch beneath the surface for this one. It is not going to get any easier the longer you ignore it. We have previously mentioned emotional abuse, and I do believe that most traumatic experiences begin with emotional abuse. Alex told me that their aunt used to take them into a room and make them get undressed. The aunt would pull out a couple of their cousin's shorts and t-shirts to try on.

Alex was not a lightweight, and their aunt, uncle, and grandparents on their dad's side would tell them that they needed to lose weight because their cousins were skinny. Alex hated going to their house, because they knew that they would be called into a room to try on some clothes and have to listen to a speech about how they needed to lose weight, have their aunt jiggle their belly flab, and listen to stories about how wonderful their cousins were. Alex grew up, but the abuse didn't stop. Instead of targeting Alex, the aunt started on their mother. The situation escalated when Alex had the opportunity to go to a tropical island for work, and the aunt was in shock because overweight Alex stayed in a luxury hotel for 10 days, went snorkeling in the ocean, and even went swimming in front of real people—flab and all! Long story short, Alex's aunt was diagnosed with cancer of the liver, and before she passed away, Alex had forgiven their aunt because they didn't want to have regrets.

No one should ever be allowed to emotionally abuse you, because you are different than others. No two people have the same body type. No two people have the same skin type. No two people are the same—*POINT!* Take a look at your fingers. Carefully examine your fingerprints. Now find someone else and examine their fingerprints. Are they the same? No, they aren't. Not even twins have the same fingerprints. Everyone on this planet has a unique fingerprint that was assigned to them the day that they were born—that was a gift that only God can give you. Why? Because you are a unique human being. Identify the hurtful situations in your life, and deal with one event at a time. Slowly, but surely, you will feel the pain lessen.

What Is the Purpose of Suffering?

This is a question I have asked myself many times. I have come up with multiple explanations, but I don't get very far before something else happens. I have heard many people, myself included, say that everything happens for a reason. Most times I can see the silver lining around the dark cloud, but many times I struggle to make sense of what is going on around me. I try my best to avoid the news, because there is so much negativity such as the rising oil prices, or a news story about a mass shooter opening fire in a public place. I avoid social media because God alone knows, if it's on social media, it is the truth and nothing but the truth—conspiracy theorists, doomsday preppers, and way too much politics to keep up with.

I was approached by someone who heard about my research and the subject I was going to write about. The elderly lady told me how she wasn't necessarily suffering, as much as she was being misused for her generosity. I listened to her story, and I realized that what was happening was indeed abuse and that this lady was suffering. Strangers, at the time, approached her and asked if they could store something on her property. They offered to pay a monthly contribution, but being the kindhearted person that she was, she told them that they could do odds and ends such as some handyman-type tasks and clearing her garden, that would be a payment. Little did the lady know that what was meant to be a temporary situation with some benefit to her, turned into a nightmare. She asked them multiple times to help her, and was dismissed and ignored. She finally plucked up the courage, sent them a message, and told them that they had two weeks to remove their stuff. She felt awful, but she had to start thinking about herself. She had been living in seclusion, because she was embarrassed to have people over, and she wanted it to end. A day and a half after giving the notice, they were at her home and clearing her property.

We stack our problems on top of each other to avoid confrontations. It is easier just to pile it on, until you reach a point that you build up so much anger that it ends in threats. You shouldn't stack your negative feelings on top of each other, because they are not hurting anyone else. You are the one that is suffering. You believe, and have been led to believe, that whatever has happened is your responsibility. For any type of healing to take place, you have to stop piling on everything that is preventing you from living your life—you have to stop taking responsibility for those who continuously disrespect you, and stand up for what is right.

Chapter 5:

Establishing Boundaries to Protect Yourself

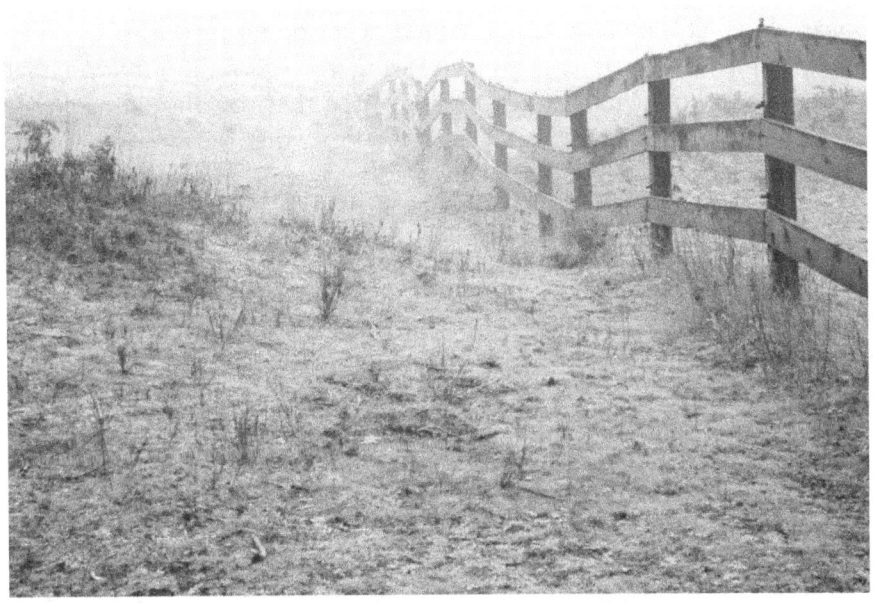

Welcome to Boundary Island. Please feel free to set down your jumbo-sized suitcase, have a seat, and take a well-deserved breather. You survived one of the most difficult islands on this island-hopping cruise. I am excited about this chapter, because it is beneficial to people of all ages, walks of life, and genders. I spoke to my editor and my publisher about this chapter before I drew up the outline, and we were all in agreement that everyone needs to be taught about boundaries. I know that many people will sit up in their chairs, or have a jaw-dropping moment when they see the importance of establishing boundaries. Please take note that this chapter is not intended to shame anyone or indicate that you are, or may be, a bad parent or caregiver. What some may see as innocence may not feel that way to you or your young children.

Everyone has a gut feeling, an intuition, or an annoying voice in your head yelling at you to be careful. The voice in your head may well drive you crazy. The secret here is not to engage in a conversation or an argument with the voices, because that will earn you a one-way ticket to a remote island—if you know what I mean. I'm just kidding, but I can tell you that I have the most intelligent conversations with the voices in my head. They keep me on my toes, they alert me when they detect red flags, and they look out for me. Something else that my voices do is let me know that I should never doubt myself or listen to the manipulators. It is easy to ignore the voices or the intuition that something is not right. I am here to tell you that you should probably listen to the voices, because 99% of the time, they know what is best for you. The other 1% most likely wants to see the look on people's faces when you're talking to yourself at the store.

Understanding the Purpose of Boundaries

- Is having boundaries a requirement in your life?

- What is the purpose of setting boundaries?

- Why are boundaries important?

I keep going back to the beginning stages of our lives. I find myself thinking about children, especially babies and toddlers, who are outgoing and trust everyone. They will go up to strangers and give their hugs away freely, or stare at them in awe. Babies and toddlers don't know about boundaries. They can't tell their parents or caregivers that they don't feel comfortable. I have noticed that when a toddler reaches the age of three, they go into that 'shy' phase where they hide behind their parents or caregivers, or even behind their hands. They are reluctant to go to strangers, family members, or friends. I do believe that this is when their gut feeling starts setting in and they start establishing personal boundaries. I think that it is at this stage that the boundaries are altered or broken down, because children are being forced to do something their gut feeling was protecting them from. I am talking about forcing them to hug someone they don't want to or kiss someone who gives sloppy kisses.

I spoke to someone whose uncle recently passed away, and she told me that she loved him very much. He was like a big brother to her, because they were so close in age. When he finished school and joined the army, she was heartbroken. When the whole family got together to take him to the train station, everyone gave him hugs, kisses, and buckets full of tears. She remembers that she never liked kissing him or hugging him, even though she loved him. Everyone forced her to hug and kiss him. She remembers him looking at her, giving her a big smile, and saying thank you. She didn't understand it at the time, and only realized the true meaning of his actions very later in life. She never stopped loving her uncle, and slept in his bed whenever she went to visit her grandmother. He got married, had a child, got divorced, traveled for work, supported her when her mother died, and they became inseparable as they only had each other. They both realized early on in their lives that they didn't like people forcing them to do things that they didn't want to do. He wasn't comfortable with people showing him any affection. He had no problem with writing or talking about affection, but it was that personal boundary that protected both of them.

The Importance of Boundaries

I have spoken about the invisible cage of protection we have ourselves trapped in. The invisible cage is a way to protect everyone from negative situations and experiences, as well as the harsh judgment, condemnation, and bullying of people. We are currently working on helping you work through, and understand, that you don't need an invisible cage. The cage is doing more harm than good, and you are being suffocated by your fears or whatever is holding you back. The blueprints I discussed in Chapter 4 were preparing you for this point, the one where you are going to learn about the importance of having boundaries. We are halfway through this journey of learning how to forgive and find the peace that we deserve.

I am going to assist you in busting out of your invisible cage. No one should be living in fear, nor should they be trapped in a cage that is suffocating them. I am going to show you what your options are, and give you some tips that you could use to custom-design your boundaries based on your requirements. Now, remember that I'm not going to tell you how you should design your boundaries. Whatever I am sharing are suggestions; you can add to what I am saying, or you can omit whatever doesn't apply. Some people may find it easier than others to set up boundaries. I will be the first to admit that establishing boundaries is hard work. It is not your intention to offend people by establishing personal boundaries.

Boundaries are established by individuals who want to protect themselves from many different types of situations. Having boundaries is vitally important to everyone. They are the rules in your personal rule book. You get to draw the invisible line around you. People will try their best to test your boundaries, and you have every right to push back. All boundaries have to be respected for your safety, and for whoever is testing them. Come on, let's start working on freeing you from your invisible cage.

The Different Types of Boundaries You Need to Establish

You are armed and ready to proceed with your blueprints. You take the first step into the maze of your life. This is not an ordinary maze that is going to lead you to dead-ends, make you backtrack, and find the right way to claim your prize. Oh no, this is a very special maze. Each 'roadblock' you encounter is going to represent boundaries. You can design as many boundaries as you need. The thing I love about establishing boundaries is knowing that I can alter them as my situation changes. I also know that I can add provisional boundaries, if I need them, by labeling them for future use. You never know when boundaries may come in handy, so it is always better to be prepared.

Physical Boundaries

My publisher, editor, and I were speaking about how boundaries have been altered. The reference at the beginning of the chapter was about babies and toddlers learning about their boundaries. We all know that it confuses people of all ages—you are told that you don't have to do anything you don't want to, but the next time you are being told, "Stop being rude, go and kiss Uncle Joe." The confusion comes in because "Uncle Joe" may not be a relative, and you don't feel comfortable hugging—much less kissing—him. I recall a time in my life when I was about six years of age, and went to the neighbor's house with my dad. The man of the house wouldn't allow me into the house without giving him a hug and a kiss. I remember that I didn't want to have any physical contact with him because he wasn't family. He said he would give me a dollar if I hugged and kissed him. After much coaxing and bribery, I did what was asked, but I didn't like it. It never felt right.

I believe that experience is possibly where my boundaries were altered and damaged. Please don't get me wrong—I am affectionate, and I love people, but the voices in my head scream when certain members of my family or friends enter my personal space. My publisher, editor, and I all agree that we do not, and would never, force our children to ignore their intuitions. We want to teach our children that they have a choice, and it is their right to want to be safe. Message to the moms and dads reading this: don't force or bribe your children to hug, kiss, or show any affection to someone they don't want to—regardless of whether they are family or not. Here is a short list of the 'rules' for the physical boundaries:

- it is your body, and you are allowed to protect it
- it is your space, and you are in control of who is allowed to cross the boundary
- it is your right to have privacy
- it is your right to eat and sleep
- it is your right to let others know your expectations

- it is your right to demand respect

Sexual Boundaries

Every relationship should begin with an open and honest discussion about each party's expectations. What we see on the television or in movies, or read in romance novels, does not portray real-life situations. It is an unrealistic expectation that you are going to meet someone while waiting in line to see your favorite band, and end up in his or her bed. Please don't come at me with your pitchforks, because I know people do this, but I am saying that not everyone does it. A relationship is built around trust, respect, and boundaries that will protect both parties. The parties have to be on the same page, because if one person is hesitant, the other party can be accused of sexual assault. I'm not saying that you need to sign a contract, but you have to have boundaries. The boundaries will include being honest about:

- both party's sexual history
- both party's sexual health
- your likes and dislikes
- your expectations

Emotional and Mental Boundaries

I have found that, out of all the boundaries that we can design, this might be the most difficult. This section is what I base all my books around. I set boundaries when I'm working on the outlines for my books. From the very beginning, when I start writing, I tell my readers about my expectations for them. I am constantly reminding my readers that this book is their safe space. I let them know that they are protected from all negativity, judgment, bullying, and whatever else they face in their daily lives. Everyone needs to feel like they have a place where they won't be mentally or emotionally hurt. I feel very strongly about protecting people. I have seen so much pain etched on people's faces when they share their stories with me, and it pains me. I have seen the effects of what a global pandemic, a senseless war for the sake of power, and unnecessary violence have done to people. My books are a giant social-distanced, full-body-armored, and peace-filled hug to everyone in need of happiness.

Don't ever be afraid to set emotional and mental boundaries. I know that you may be overwhelmed with this crucial design for your blueprints, but it is very important. You don't have to use your squeaky voice anymore. Reach deep into your soul, unlock the cage that has had you silenced, and let your voice be heard. Be loud and proud about your intentions, and don't hold back. Remember, you are reclaiming your life, and you have the right to demand respect from family, friends, and anyone who dares say anything negative or derogatory about you. Emotional and mental boundaries will include:

- the protection of your feelings
- the protection of your thoughts
- the protection against being victimized
- that you are not responsible for other people
- respecting other people's privacy
- respecting other people's feelings, even when they don't respect you
- not allowing people to take away your voice

Roundup

I touched on some of the most important boundaries that I felt were manipulated or ignored the most. I am not, under any circumstances, saying that other boundaries are not important. ALL boundaries are important, and this helps everyone. I cannot stress the importance of boundaries enough. It is both healing for people who have and are experiencing trauma, as well as those who are victims of being taken advantage of. Remember that the blueprints can be added to, or amended, as needed. What you are seeing is an example of what you could implement to your circumstances. Other types of boundaries I did not mention include:

- spiritual
- religious
- financial

The Benefits of Boundaries

I have shared why it is important to have boundaries. I want everyone to have a chance to stake their place in this world. I have seen too many people get burned by others disrespecting established boundaries. What can you expect from yourself by setting boundaries? Do you get a gift card from your favorite soda shop? Do you get a free scratch card? Unfortunately, you do not get an award, a monetary reward, or anything of value in the real world. However, you will receive peace of mind, happiness, and a very reduced load on the luggage you haul around on your shoulders. Everything you do, from here on out, is to your advantage, and to strengthen your mental, emotional, and physical health and well-being. My biggest wish for you when establishing boundaries, and putting yourself first, is that you will believe in yourself, never give up fighting for your rights, and never have to settle for anything less than the best.

Setting Yourself up for Success

I cannot stress enough the importance of boundaries in one's life. I have witnessed how people are bullied because they are afraid to stand up for themselves. I know that you don't want to live in that invisible cage any longer. I know that you want to have the chance to forgive people so that you can move on with your life. I realize that you may not be ready to put your plan of forgiveness into action just yet, but you are approaching that pedestal. I am just here, in the background, offering you the guidance and giving you the confidence, to break out of your invisible cage. What do I get out of helping you set up boundaries, and teaching you about forgiving people who hurt you?

Absolutely nothing but sincere happiness. Let's inspect a couple of the benefits you could look forward to when establishing boundaries.

Control Over Emotions

You know that burning feeling that you get in the pit of your stomach—no, not indigestion! The burning that makes your blood boil, and all you see and feel is anger, rage, and hatred? That feeling will begin to fade when you start establishing boundaries. You are in charge of the feelings inside you. It is up to you to let everyone know that they have to follow any rules and regulations about your life. You are allowed to let people know that you will not tolerate anyone bullying or taking advantage of your good nature. Remember that you do need to communicate the terms of your boundaries. You can give people a three-strike warning, and on the last strike, they have a choice. I like to believe that everything in life is about giving people choices. It is safe to say that once you have let people know how you feel, you will not need any antacids to cool that burning feeling.

Bathed in Tranquility and Serenity

There is nothing better than waking up in the morning feeling as light as a feather. This is what everyone needs to aim for in their life. It is a great feeling to know that, after sharing the terms and conditions of your boundaries, you are protected. It may take a while before you are comfortably enjoying the tranquility and serenity you have been dreaming of. I know that it is hard to change old habits. I know that you will shuffle around, looking over your shoulder in fear. I know that it is just a matter of time until you realize that you don't have to hide in your invisible cage anymore. That will be the moment when you know and understand that you have reached the top of your boundary of empowerment—compassion.

Another one of the beautiful takeaways from setting boundaries is that you start experiencing new feelings. You may have been hiding behind your fear, or hardened your heart to protect yourself. The crusty and hardened exterior vanishes the moment you set clear and definitive boundaries. You have told everyone the dos and don'ts about your boundaries, and that in itself is a massive groundbreaking moment in your life. You will feel as if you have been knocked off your perch, your invisible cage is gone, and you feel like a new person. You will start having new, alien-like feelings that you have never felt before. You will see people who have hurt you through a new lens. That is what compassion is all about.

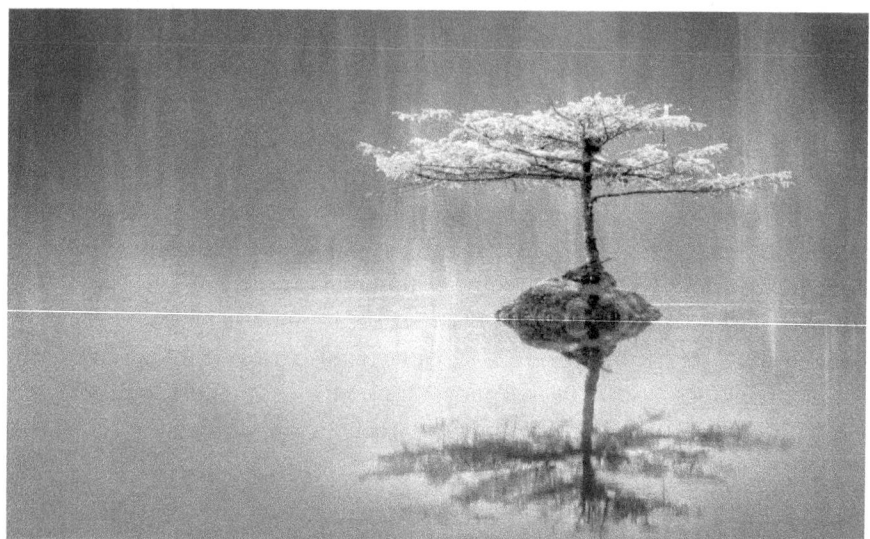

Chapter 6:

Learning How to Let Go of Grudges

This may be the chapter everyone needs to read. I believe that everyone holds onto grudges or bitterness. Human beings are a unique breed of individuals, and I say that with much love and affection, as well as bemusement and anger. I have previously mentioned that no two people are alike, which is what makes everyone unique. Everyone has traits and quirks that get on people's nerves. If someone does something that you don't like, you don't say anything, but you stick it in a compartment in your memory for future use. The next time that you see that person, you scratch around for the memory, and you end up scrutinizing the person and may even call them out on something they did three years previously. You may recall that I spoke about the fact that as much as you want, you cannot change the past. I hold strong in that belief. Why would you, me, or anyone else want to hold onto something that can't be changed? We end up wasting precious hours, energy, and emotions on what happened—when we could have been focusing on building relationships with family, friends, and loved ones, or taking care of ourselves.

We set out on a cruise that would take us to 10 different islands. The goal of the cruise was to free you from the clutches of the past. You have spent half of this cruise lugging around a suitcase that is filled with past hurt, negativity, judgment, condemnation, and trauma. As we prepare to step onto the next leg of our journey together, I would like to make a suggestion that may be beneficial to you. The next couple of islands we will be visiting are more about discovering what is best for you. I showed you how to set boundaries and why they were beneficial to your mental, emotional, and physical well-being. I believe that, going forward, your suitcase is protected by the boundaries you have established. You have done everything you could to protect yourself from any pain or trauma from your past. It is my wish that you will continue this journey without any burdens. I want to show you how you can let go of grudges or bitterness, and discover what you have missed out on. I am also going to share some handy tips and tricks to help you forgive people. I have previously touched on some of the hints, but a refresher is always a good idea, as it will help soothe your rising anxiety levels.

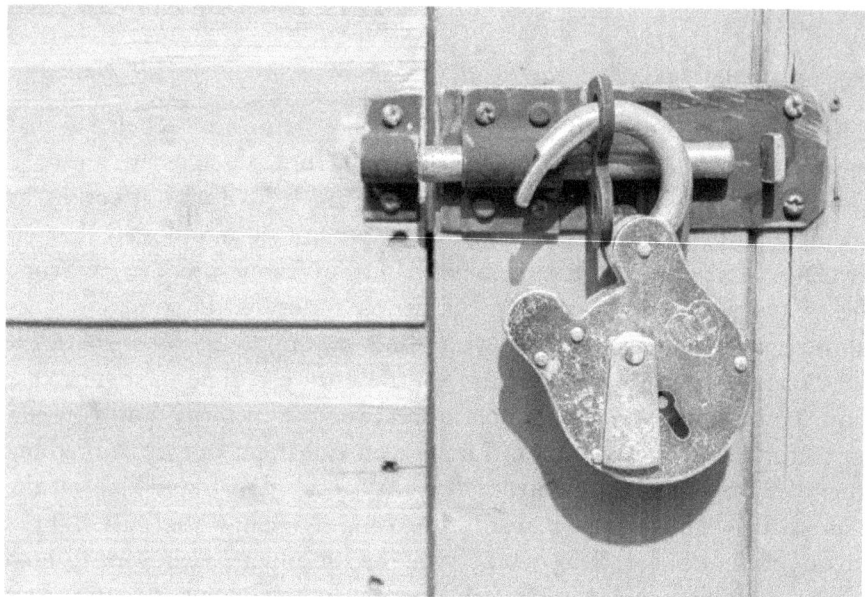

Signs That You Are Holding a Grudge

At what point in your life do you think about why you don't want to speak to someone, or go somewhere? This is something that I have had to think about, because I was experiencing strange feelings whenever a name, a place, or something came up in conversation. I interviewed a lady who had the same type of experience as me. This lady was incredibly difficult to read. The look in her eyes was that of someone who was deeply guarded in shame. She started telling me about her experience in high school, and how she was bullied by classmates, teachers, and faculty members. Every couple of days, the faculty members would call her out for something stupid like her shoes were not shining, she wasn't wearing her blazer, or her socks weren't turned down properly. Her classmates, especially the girls, were nasty and played horrible pranks on her. They jeered at her, or the boys would accidentally walk into her and touch her inappropriately. She spoke to the guidance counselor, who brushed her off.

One day, one of her classmates lost her contact lenses, and everyone went on a scavenger hunt to find the case. She remembers going into the bathroom to look, when two of her classmates walked in behind her. The lady found the contact lens kit, and was leaving the bathroom to return it to the girl. Instead of her returning it, the two classmates snatched it from her hands, and hightailed it out of the bathrooms to return it themselves. They received all the praise. She was heartbroken, and not because she wanted the praise and recognition—she just wanted everyone to see that she was a nice person.

A couple of days after the incident, the girl whose contact lenses went missing handed the two classmates a reward—a gift bag filled with threats. This made the lady angry, because the two flaunted the bags around and even 'accidentally' bumped into her with them. Then she did something she was, and is, not proud of. When the classmates were at phys ed, she happened to be called into the principal's office for something; and when she left, she went past the lockers, and stole one of the gift bags. When the classmates discovered that the one gift bag was missing, they went to the teacher, who made all the girls stay after class. She told them to step away from their school bags, and initiated a search. Naturally, the lady was first, but she had been clever, and stashed the gift bag elsewhere.

For the first time in her life, a teacher stood up for her, and told her classmates that they shouldn't blame people without evidence. The lady felt guilty, but she had wanted to teach her classmates a lesson. She went back to the hiding place after school, hid the items from the gift bag in her school bag, and went home. She says that she did indulge in some of the candy treats, but she also gave candy to the kids in the neighborhood. The lady never had a problem with her grade that year, because her parents had decided it would be best for her to repeat a year at school because of the trauma of bullying. As for the candy and the classmates—she never admitted her thievery to anyone, but she also knew that the two classmates knew that it was her and she didn't care. Many years later, she ran into one of her classmates who couldn't wait to tell everyone who listened to her what she had done—including her pastor.

Inspecting the Root of Grudges

The lady knows that she has to seek forgiveness for what she had done, but she doesn't want to see those classmates because of how they treated her. I asked her if she still had a grudge against them, and she said, without even thinking, that she had a grudge against everyone who bullied her. No one ever told her that they were sorry, and she has been holding onto that pain for many years. I asked her again if she was planning to meet them face-to-face? She shook her head and said that she was in the process of reshaping her life. She said that she was facing some difficult obstacles, which include asking for forgiveness, and forgiving others. She did say that she was not prepared to step outside of her boundaries just to break down all the work she had put into her healing. She was not going to make herself vulnerable, because she went through five years of relentless bullying.

There are any number of things that can lead to the point where we build up years' worth of anger, hatred, and resentment. The human mind is a mysterious part of the body. I often find myself thinking about where everything I see, read, or hear is stored in my brain. I am in awe of people who can remember every detail of their childhood. I am even more amazed when people remember everything that others have done to hurt them. More often than not, people do remember all the things that have had a negative impact on their lives. It is much easier to stack your dislikes and build up resentment toward a person, or circumstances. It is even more convenient to sweep everything under the mat where it becomes a "toxic dumpsite." That is what we are doing to ourselves. We are allowing this toxicity to seep into our daily lives. We have built up an immunity to this toxicity without even realizing it. We need to sort through the compartments in our minds, and get rid of grudges. I know that you are cursing, and most likely saying, "over my dead body," but this is something that will help you going forward.

You can't please everyone. I know that, you know that, and everyone else knows it too. You can try, yes, but you will end up being hurt and your toxic dumpsite will grow bigger. Something that each one of us can do, is take a small leap of faith to make our world—not the entire world—a better place. We can spread the healing and positivity to others when we have become the masters and mistresses of our little worlds. I can't recall if I have mentioned it before, but I am an eternal optimist, and I like to see the good in everyone. That is why I believe that positive changes start with one person, and spread to others; and before you know it, people from all across the globe will experience the positive effects of getting rid of the toxic dumpsite.

Inspecting Our Toxic Dumpsites

We are going to sort through your toxic dumpsite to uncover what you may have swept under the mat. Here you may just learn that you have been harboring grudges that mean nothing to anybody other than your pride. This is an important part of healing. You want people to respect the boundaries that you have set, but you aren't willing to seek forgiveness for something you have done. This is where the gears shift, and I point out what holding onto grudges looks like. Together we are going to take a quick rummage through the dumpsite to see what types of triggers we can find. Remember my rules—open minds, nonjudgmental, free of condemnation, and a new addition of letting go of grudges you don't need.

The Manipulation Associated With Grudges

Grudges are master manipulators that sneak in and fill your mind with different renditions unrelated to the actual problem. I have found that most people aren't aware that they have been harboring a grudge against someone. We are all victims of the grudges that are sneakily implanted in our minds. You may be doing something one moment, and the next you are experiencing extreme frustration. There is nothing worse than being frustrated about something and not knowing where that frustration originated from.

Someone once told me that grudges were designed to bring unnecessary conflict to our lives. I was also told that if you can't remember any incidents, then it was never important, and you should probably let it go. I would make a bet that when you go through your suitcase, you can remove at least half of what you are carrying around. This is your time to shine, and you have the power to release those grudges into the ocean.

Making Sure That Your Voice Is Heard

You were introduced to Alex in Chapter 2. They had so many stories and so much wisdom related to the topic of this book, that I had to include their experiences. Alex was the type of person everyone would go to for advice or a dose of positivity. They didn't like confrontation, which opened them up to people taking advantage of their good nature. Alex didn't know how to use the word, *no*. They tried, but it always seemed to evaporate into thin air. They always ended up giving in and doing what others asked, told, or demanded of them.

Alex knew that they had built up a pretty decent toxic dumpsite. They collected and held onto everything that people would say or do to them. Alex built up a lot of resentment toward people who continually took advantage of them, until one day when everybody got a piece of their mind. Alex told me that they wrote a four-page Word document. The document consisted of the names of all the people who had been bleeding the stone dry. They didn't hold back in their writing. Alex explained that they had just reached the boiling point. They had decided that everyone needed to be informed at the same time. Each of the names had a message attached, explaining why Alex felt the way they did. Alex then ended the letter by saying that their boundaries had been ignored and disrespected. Everyone mentioned received a three-strike penalty. They could earn their way back if they showed Alex respect, and treated them the way they wanted others to treat them.

Alex wants everyone, whether victims or instigators, to know that they should use their voices. All the corners in all the houses or buildings are full—no one should be hiding in the corners.

Moving on and Letting Go

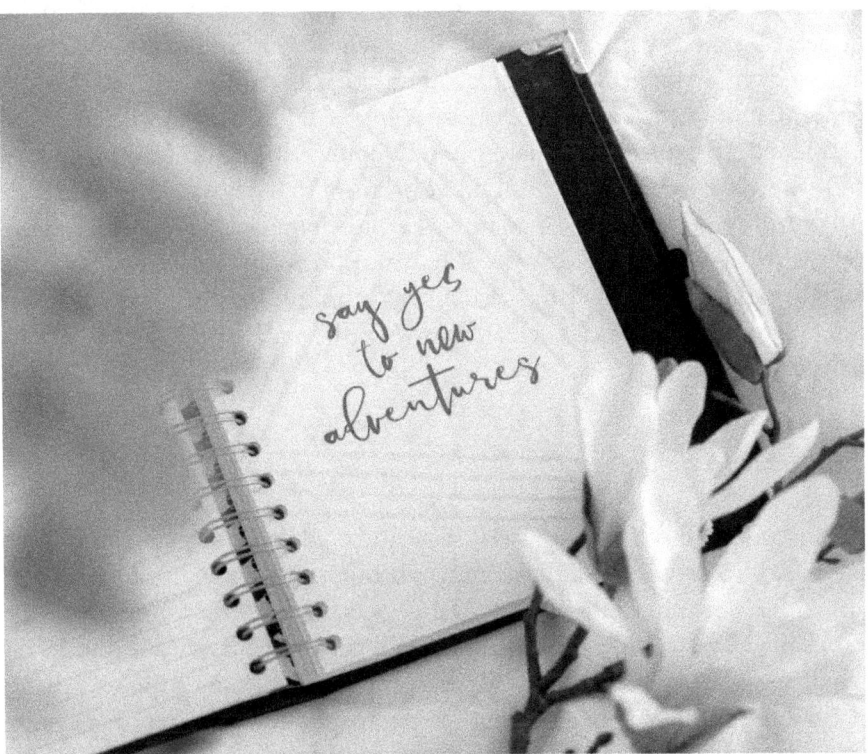

You know that it is time to clear your toxic dumpsite. I also know that you are hesitant, because you are afraid to let go of your security blanket. You are looking at the grudges you have gathered over the years, and you are contemplating which ones you want to keep. Holding onto grudges has become a habit. You know, as well as I do, that you can't change what has happened. All that you are doing is holding onto something that is making you a bitter and angry person, and quite possibly affecting your health.

- Do you want to live the rest of your life filled with bitterness?

- Are you afraid to let go of your grudges?

- Would you consider letting go of grudges, and replacing them with positive thoughts and affirmations?

These are just a few questions that you can ask yourself. The yes/no questions are neither right, nor wrong. You owe it to yourself to be honest, because you are the only one who is suffering. No one else knows why you are carrying around moldy grudges. I can almost guarantee that the person you are angry with has forgotten what happened. I have previously shared some tips, but I do think a refresher is always welcome. Did you know that you are the gardener of your life? It's true, because only *you* can shape your life. You are the one who has to get rid of weeds, harmful bugs, and overgrowth. Let's take a look at some helpful gardening techniques to help your garden repair from the drought, clear away weeds, and install a water-wise irrigation system.

Journaling

This is one of my favorite ways to get through the obstacles that hold me back. I believe that journaling has brought me to where I am today, an author of multiple books. Many people find that writing is an excellent way to wade through your innermost feelings. Writing down whatever is in your heart and mind is part of the healing process. I have previously spoken about writing letters to people who may have hurt you, or who you needed to ask for forgiveness. I also said that you didn't have to send those letters if you didn't want to, and that you could burn them and release the negativity that has been holding you back.

Journaling will help you find the peace you are longing for. You may remember more about a particular incident the moment your pen hits the paper. I have found that people who journal don't like speaking about themselves. They are very reserved, and don't want to be a burden to others. I know that journaling may not be for everyone, but I am positive that everyone will find something that works for them, and helps them find a happy medium to get rid of what is holding them back.

Changing Perspective

Something I may have spoken about previously was taking a step back and acknowledging the situation, experience, or person you have a grudge against. This is a practice that may be difficult for many people. Throughout this book, I have been protecting you as best I possibly can. I may have pushed you here and there so that you could see what things look like from the other side. I have respected your boundaries, but now I am going to ask you to shift the way you view a difficult situation. I will still be protecting you, and your boundaries will remain intact.

You need to change places with the people you have a grudge against. Take a look at the world through their eyes. Replay the situation in your mind, and see if you can find the point where they either intentionally or accidentally hurt you. What did they do for you to harden your heart and fill you with anger? Did they criticize your parenting skills? Did they hurt your feelings by saying that they didn't like the color of your dress? Did they perhaps say something about the food you are eating? Is it possible that you misunderstood the context of what they were saying? Is it possible that you didn't like where the conversation was going?

I cannot stress it enough that we live in a world where the rules we had 50 years ago have been drastically altered. Yes, rules do change; and yes, it is important for growth. I believe that we have reached the time and space where even the rules have rules. You only have to watch the news on the television, click a link to a reputable news agency, or listen to the radio to know how people are feeling. We are surrounded by negativity; and unfortunately, we absorb it, and implement it in our own lives. We are quick to jump to conclusions, we are quick to pass judgment, and we are extremely quick to blame someone for something they didn't realize they were doing. In short, we are not giving anyone the time to backtrack and make amends for what they have done.

Roundup

Do you want to continue holding a grudge against someone, or are you ready to let it wash away with the ebb and flow of the tide? This is a question only you can answer. You have to reevaluate your life, and reach a place where you can and will be happy. What better place to start, than by doing what everyone's favorite Disney princess has been doing since 2013, which is—Let It Go! Wipe the slate clean by:

- acknowledging the anger that you have against someone

- accepting what happened, as well as understanding that you can't change what happened

- bundling up the hurt, anger, rage, or regret, and tossing it in the ocean—preferably far away from land

- adopting positivity into your life

- being the person that you want to be, and not the person circumstances demand that you should be

Chapter 7:

Utilizing Alternative Practices to Ease the Journey to Forgiveness

Welcome to the island of Zen. This is where I am going to tell you that it is a requirement to leave your suitcase (lighter load) on the cruise ship. This is not a bullying or strategic tactic to force you to do something that you don't want to do. We have explored many nooks and crooks on the islands we have visited. You learned how to set boundaries, how to deal with grudges, and how to take care of yourself. The knowledge you have gained has taken you outside of your comfort zone. Your anxiety levels were fluctuating more than the exchange rates of foreign currencies. I believe that you are ready to piece together everything you have learned to make positive changes in your life.

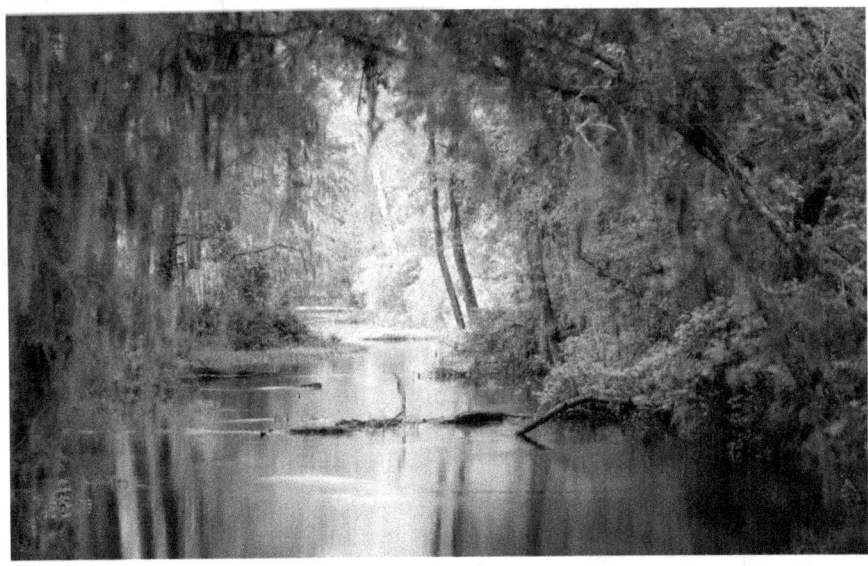

I would like to remind you that I am not a therapist or a medical professional. I am not here to give you any medical advice, and whatever I share is what works for me. If you have any concerns or queries about your mental health, I strongly suggest that you seek the help of a medical professional. Do not go to the *Medical Practice of Google*. While many may believe that Dr. Google has all the answers, I can assure you that whatever you are presently researching would have put you in the grave five years ago. Your mental, physical, and emotional health and well-being are important to your family, loved ones, and quite possibly the cashier at the local Target who looks forward to your smile whenever you go to the store.

This chapter is about finding alternative or holistic methods—which do not include the use of herbs, supplements, or medication—to help people deal with trauma, stress, or anxiety related to dealing with painful memories. At no point during this chapter will I tell you to go out and face those who hurt you. This chapter will be a "behind the scenes" healing practice that will be beneficial to helping you find the peace you need and deserve. I previously mentioned that you cannot expect to be better in the blink of an eye. I don't believe in quick fixes when it comes to one's self-care. This is not a process you can rush. It is true that some people may experience changes quicker than others, but healing from something is not a race. Healing is not a process that can be rushed, and it will take more patience and perseverance than you ever thought possible to achieve the desired goal at the end of the day.

Self-Healing Techniques That Work

The idea behind self-healing is not taking two Tylenol, and crawling into bed. Self-healing is something that everyone should be doing to take care of themselves. The list of self-healing ideas is endless. This is one of those lists that you can't really get wrong, because you are encouraged to do things that make you feel good about yourself. When someone is starting a new lifestyle program, they are told to incorporate exercise into their lives. Many people don't like going to the gym, or they don't like people staring them down when they're walking around the neighborhood. Everyone has a home gym in their sitting rooms, kitchen pantries, and even the garden. Grab a vacuum cleaner, a broom, or a mop and start cleaning. Grab a couple of cans from the pantry, place them in two plastic bags, and work on your arms. Struggling with insomnia? Don't worry, self-help tips are aplenty. You are not here to learn about diet, exercise, and lack of sleep. You are here to learn some techniques that will help your anxiety, and ease you through the jungle that is the barrier between yourself and forgiveness.

I am going to share a couple of techniques to help you on your road to healing, and eventually forgiveness. You may not yield any results after one or two days of following these practices. I don't want to lead you around by the nose and fill you with expectations for immediate results. I have a moral contract with myself to always be honest. This is part of the boundaries that I have set for myself. Remember, I know why you are on this journey, and I know how you may be feeling. I have an army behind me, who are on the same journey, and they can tell you that it is an ongoing process. They will possibly even tell you that anyone who advertises quick fixes for anything, is sniffing their socks. And truth be told—if there were quick fixes, I would likely pass on by and continue with the longer reward, because I would want to work out all the kinks and enjoy the reward at the end of it.

Forgiveness Technique: An Ancient Hawaiian Mantra

I was introduced to the Hawaiian mantra, the *Ho'oponopono Prayer*, by my publisher who shared that this was something they had implemented into their daily life. Naturally curious, I had turned to my research assistant, Professor Google, to do a little investigating. I came across an article titled, *The Hawaiian Secret of Forgiveness: Ho'oponopono can help anyone let go of resentment*, that was penned by Dr. Matt James, Ph.D., for the online publication *Psychology Today*. The article focuses on the lessons that we need to learn to practice forgiving others. Doctor James explains that when people practice the ho'oponopono, they are initiating the healing process by severing the connection they may have to the people who hurt them. In essence, you are learning how to clear that toxic dumpsite we mentioned earlier. Before you can add anything clean and positive to your life, you must clean the old (James, 2011).

The Ho'oponopono Prayer

This Hawaiian practice is not a religious prayer. Some people refer to it as a mantra or chant, as they only repeat the four phrases. The ho'oponopono prayer is made up of four very powerful phrases. Each of the phrases represents an area in your life that needs healing or affirmation, such as asking for forgiveness and mercy, and expressing love and thanks. Most people find it difficult to practice any one of the four areas, and this prayer is asking you to incorporate them all into one mantra. Okay, I can sense that you are holding your breath, so slowly exhale and breathe in lungs full of fresh air. This practice does not require you to face anyone that has been or currently is causing you pain by their words, action, or deeds.

I have been told that this ho'oponopono prayer could dredge up some memories you may not want to deal with. The idea behind this mantra is that you focus on the person, people, or situation that hurt you. Say you have an infected wound on your body... It would be easy to put some cream on it, slap on a Band-Aid, and off you go. Two days later, the wound is not healing and you end up at the doctor's office because the wound has started festering. The doctor asks you what you used on your wound, and you tell them the name of the cream. The doctor asks a couple more questions, and eventually tells you that the wound won't get better because you didn't properly clean it. The doctor sterilizes the wound, cleans it out, uses an antibiotic ointment, and bandages it up. They give you a list of instructions on what you need to do to take care of the wound at home. The ho'oponopono prayer is your instruction list for healing your mind, body, and soul.

- I am sorry.
- (Please) Forgive me.
- Thank you.
- I love you.

Four very powerful phrases may help you find the peace you need to move forward with your life. Everything I researched about the ho'oponopono prayers indicates that you don't have to say these phrases in any particular order for them to be effective. Trust and allow your instinct to lead you through this process. I have tried to find an example of how you can use this prayer, but I have failed. The phrases are so powerful that they don't need examples. The more you say them, the more you learn about yourself, and relish in the healing that it comes with. I will, however, share what I have been doing, which has worked very well for me.

I have written each of the phrases on multiple sticky notes. I walked through my home and put them everywhere that they would stick on such as my refrigerator, microwave oven, and all the mirrors I could find. I do believe any guests would think I have lost my way to Sanityville, but my mental health and well-being are more important than what other people think. The sticky notes are a constant reminder that healing is part of the journey to finding peace by forgiving. The sticky notes remind me of where I have been, where I am, and where I am going. Before I go to sleep at night, I incorporate the ho'oponopono prayer into my nightly conversation with God. I say sorry to anyone I may have hurt by something I did or said. I ask for forgiveness, as well as forgive those who have hurt me in any way, shape, or form. I thank everyone for all the blessings and lessons I learned that day. And I always end off with an, "I love you," to the universe because I have so much love in me that I know I can share it with those who are struggling to find love.

Forgiveness Technique: Meditation

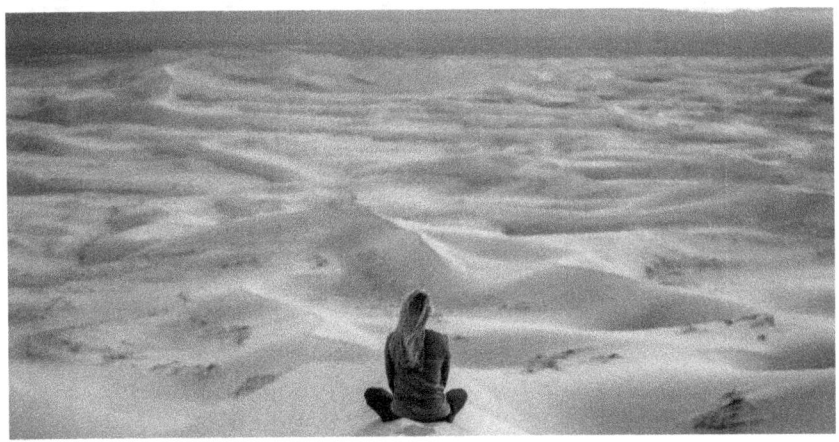

The following technique is one that originated in India, and was practiced by Hindus and Buddhists. These selfless spiritualists didn't keep their techniques locked behind closed doors, and they shared their practices with everyone who would listen. Meditation is an excellent technique that is used to manage stress or anxiety which could negatively impact your life. We become so caught up in the rat race known as life, that we neglect our physical, mental, and emotional health. I like the idea of incorporating meditation into my daily life, because it reminds me to take 10 minutes out of a busy day to focus on myself.

I know that meditation is something that people from all walks of life don't believe in. I find myself trying to understand why people would find it necessary to criticize something that they have been practicing without realizing the origin. I am a deeply spiritual person, but I am also very open-minded. I am not going to run someone else's beliefs into the ground because I don't agree with them. I practice yoga and meditation, which essentially is exercise and breathing. We are so caught up in trying to do everything according to the 'rules,' that we forget that nobody is forced to choose this way or that. Everything that we do in life has to originate somewhere. I'm sure that whichever religion you believe in, you will be forgiven for doing something that will benefit your health and well-being.

According to an article written by the Mayo Clinic Staff, the practice of meditation has many benefits to one's overall mental, physical, and emotional well-being. Please feel free, dear skeptics, to take on medical professionals who use an ancient practice to help people:

- see what stress can do
- manage their stress
- realize that they are worthy
- realize that they don't have to live in the past
- eliminate the negative energy that they have locked away
- lower their resting blood pressure and/or heart rate

- rest peacefully

- eliminate headaches

- reduce depression

- cope with anxiety

Types of Meditation

The Mayo Clinic Staff article also shares a list of different meditation practices. I wanted to share this list with you, so that you could see their names. I do believe that yoga, and mindful and guided meditation, are the most popular practices. As I have previously mentioned, these ancient meditation practices have been used by billions of people from all walks of faith. They may just have been hiding behind different names. Can I share a secret with you? God doesn't mind if you do yoga, tai chi, or guided meditation. How do I know? You'll have to wait until Chapters 8 and 9 to find out.

- yoga

- tai chi

- qigong

- mantra meditation

- mindfulness meditation

- guided meditation

Preparing for Meditation

It doesn't matter which type of meditation practice you choose. The principles of meditation, which I will introduce to you here, stay the same. There may be an addition here or there, but it is up to the person practicing to do what is best for them.

- Find a quiet place.

- Get yourself into a comfortable position by either sitting on the floor, on a chair, on the bed, or laying on the floor or the bed.

- Have an open mind.

- Block out sounds and distractions.

- Focus on yourself.

- Practice breathing—in through the nose, out through the mouth.

These steps are just the beginning of a more peaceful life. Remember that learning the ins and outs, and implementing the tools for meditation, is going to require you to practice patience. It is hard work, especially when you don't know how to turn the focus to yourself. You may have become so self-conscious that you don't want to put yourself in the spotlight, even if you are the one being showcased. You are not practicing meditation for anyone other than yourself. This is your journey, which I have told you many times, to learn how to forgive and claim back your life (Mayo Clinic Staff, 2022).

Example of a Meditation Session

I wanted to give you an example of what a meditation session may look like. I tried to find a basic scripted meditation that you could customize to suit your preferences. Goodness, that was a difficult task. I listened to many different meditations until I found one that I thought would be ideal for beginners. You will find the website in the reference section, and I will give all the credit for the inspiration to Paul Harrison, who is a meditation teacher. I have to insert another warning here to the skeptics—no, this is not some type of mind control activity (Harrison, 2021).

1. The most important part of the meditation journey is that you have to leave your device in another room. You are going to do this without any distractions.

2. Find a quiet place, and get comfortable.

3. Close your eyes, take a couple of moments, and allow yourself to relax.

4. Next, you are going to pay close attention to your breathing. Breathe in through your nose for 5 counts, and exhale through your mouth for 5 counts. Do this at least 10 times.

5. Think about the person, people, or the situation where you were traumatized or hurt.

6. Continue with your breathing as the memories start popping up. Remember that the memories cannot hurt you. Take note of thoughts you have toward those who have hurt you.

7. Keep reminding yourself that the person you are seeing cannot hurt you in your memories. You are safe, and you are protected. Breathe and keep telling yourself that memories can't hurt you. Imagine that the person you are seeing is on a piece of paper, and you are going to crumble it up, and toss it in the trash can.

8. Continue thinking about this person. What may have triggered this person to say or do something to hurt you? Are you aware that the person was having any personal problems that may have been the root cause of why they did or said what they did? Make a mental list in your mind of everything that may be an indication of the change in their attitude. Continue reminding yourself that you are in a safe place, and that the memories can't hurt you.

9. Your mental list starts producing answers. You remember when the person started changing. All the answers start adding up, and you begin to understand why they said or did what they did. You begin to see that you may have been in the wrong place, at the wrong time, and that you were collateral damage.

10. You are going to visualize the person standing in front of you. Remember that you are safe, alone, and memories can't hurt you. Tell the image standing before you that you understand what they did. Acknowledge that they caused you pain, and tell them that you forgive them.

11. You may be emotional at this point, which is normal during meditation. You are going to reach into your virtual suitcase, dig out the painful memories of what happened, and you are going to drop them in the ocean. That is how you are going to forgive this person, and walk away. You have forgiven someone for hurting you, and now that you have released that hurt, you can't take it back. The memories will be with you, but they are only carbon copies, because the originals have been destroyed. In time, the memories will begin to fade.

12. Focus on your breathing. Breathe in through your nose for 5 counts, and breathe out through your mouth for 5 counts. Continue this practice 10 times. This will help release any residual tension. When you are ready, you can open your eyes and relax, while you reflect on the mammoth task you have accomplished.

Chapter 8:

I Thought God Would Protect Me From Pain and Suffering

Welcome to the Island of Understanding. I had to think about where to put this chapter so that it wouldn't offend any of my readers who have burned the Bridge of Religion. Please believe me when I tell you that you are not human if you haven't burned the bridge a couple of times during your lifetime. Religion is a sensitive subject to people from all walks of life. In the last couple of years, after a global pandemic claimed the lives of so many, people lost their faith. The conspiracy theorists were like deer caught in headlights, as they shared their opinions with everyone. The religious fundamentalists were convinced that the end of the world was upon us, and that the rapture was imminent. Other religious groups encouraged their members to stock up on their food storage and prepare for doomsday.

This may very well be the part of this cruise that you have been dreading the most. I wanted to be respectful to all my readers, which is why I decided to wait until close to the end, to bring religion into the fold. You know that I have presented myself in a nonjudgmental and compassionate manner. I have empathy for *ALL* people, regardless of their ethnicity, gender, body type, religion, or finances. I even have empathy toward those who have hurt me, continue to hurt me, and who may hurt me in the future. I don't hate very easily, but I do get angry. When I get angry, I can't sleep, because the memories come alive. I asked God why He is allowing these memories to take my breath away, and suffocate me. Naturally, I didn't get an answer, because God put me in the cooler box to calm down. I repeated the ho'oponopono prayer a couple of times. I said that I was sorry for the way I was reacting because I was angry, asked for forgiveness, said thank you, and told Him that I loved Him.

After repeating the prayer a couple of times, I realized that God was with me because I became calmer, and fell asleep for a couple of hours. God is always with us. What He wants from us is to trust in Him. We don't see that, because we are impatient and expect everything to happen at the drop of a hat. I have been down that road one too many times, and so have you. I do believe that we were not, will not, and never will be, the only ones who have these feelings. You are allowed to ask questions. You are allowed to be angry at God or whichever deity you worship. It took me many years to understand that He will never forsake me. Something we all have to understand is that time in heaven doesn't work the same as it does on earth. A day on earth could be a second in heaven. I know that it is frustrating, but as I previously mentioned, we have to learn to trust and have a little bit of faith.

Are you ready to grab a bucket of faith, a spade of trust, and a curious person wanting to understand why things happen the way they do? I am not forcing you to change your beliefs. I am not sugarcoating anything for your reading pleasure. I know and understand that religion is a sensitive topic to many. All I have ever asked of you is that you keep an open mind. Everyone is allowed to have an opinion, but you don't have to dissuade others or fill their minds with doubt. Remember that everyone has the right to choose whatever they want without being bullied.

Crossing the Bridge of Religion

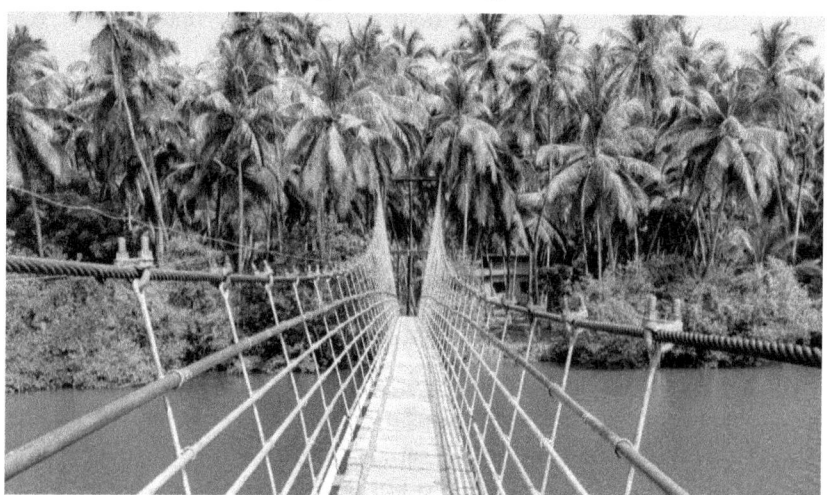

Have you ever read the comment section when watching videos on YouTube, looking at posts on Instagram, or scrolling through Facebook? I'm not ashamed to say that I find comment sections both entertaining and frustrating. I get a little hot under the collar by some of the responses, hit that reply, and type in what I want to say. Before I can enter the message, I am doused in a virtual tub of ice-cold water, and I press the backspace button to erase what I was going to say. It is part of human nature to want to defend and protect what we believe. Most people don't take the time to think about what they are saying, or who they are offending when they start spewing hurtful comments.

We are not oblivious to what goes on in the world. Everyone is exposed to multiple media publications, social media platforms, and word-of-mouth sources. One just has to observe the body language or listen to someone speak to know how they are feeling about what is happening. I think that the population can be divided into two different groups. One group of people are like ducks where the water bounces off of them. The other group of people are like sponges who absorb everything that they read, see, and are told. There is no right or wrong group to be part of, because everyone walking around on this earth adds value to being part of the population.

Why Does God Allow Suffering?

I think that the, "Where is God when we are suffering," question is one of the most asked. The answers I have seen make my heart break for those people. What happened to them to make them so hateful? Many people were raised to believe that God watches over them, and that He is always with them. I can understand the anger, resentment, and sadness when people feel that God failed them in their time of need. God understands it, too. I had someone tell me that God knows what you are going to do before the thought is planted in your mind. Someone else told me that their late mother told them that God knows the date of our death on the day that we take our first breath. God knows how we are going to die; and that if it is your time, there is no way to change what has been prophesied when you were born.

I know that many people may not agree with either of the pieces I shared, but many people hold onto these words of pearls of wisdom—

and who are you or I, to take it away from them. Everyone is free to believe whatever they want to, and it is not my place to tell you how it should be. I have had many of my interviewees ask me what my stance is when asked this question. My answer, to anyone who has ever asked, is that I am an eternal optimist who believes that things happen for a reason. Well, I can tell you that I have received a lot of backlash because of my opinion. I have had people wanting to start debates with me, and telling me that my opinions are skewed.

- Do I believe that someone is meant to be sexually abused or assaulted?

- Do I believe that someone is meant to perish at the hands of someone who has no regard for human life?

Absolutely not. It is not my place to hand down a judgment of people who do wrong in the world. I am not the judge of that person or those individuals. I do get angry. I cry with the families. I refer you to the mother who forgave her son's murderer in Chapter 2. What would you have done in her position? Lived with hatred, plot revenge on the boy and his family? What will that get you? You are going to stand before the Judge of all judges one day. You are going to answer to God when He asks you why you believed it was your duty to be the judge, jury, and executioner. Are you going to tell Him that the person you condemned never hurt you, but that you felt that it was your duty to fight for the victim? The fundamentalists will be jumping up and down while waving their pom-poms around, because the New International Version (NIV) of the Bible in Matthew 7:1–2 says: "Do not judge, or you too will be judged. For in the same way you judge others, you will be judged, and with the measure you use, it will be measured to you." Guess what? The Bible also tells us in Galatians 1:1–5: "Paul, an apostle—sent not from men nor by a man, but by Jesus Christ and God the Father, who raised him from the dead—an all the brothers and sisters with me, to the churches in Galatia: Grace and peace to you from God our Father and the Lord Jesus Christ, who gave himself for our sins to rescue us from the present evil age, according to the will of our God and Father, to whom be glory for ever and ever. Amen." As if that verse was not enough confirmation, 1 Peter 2:24 tells us that, 'He himself bore our sins," in his body on the cross, so that we might die to sins and live for righteousness; "by his wounds you have been healed."

I would like to insert a gentle reminder that this is a nonjudgmental book where everyone is allowed to have opinions. You do not, and are not required to, believe everything that is being said—but I do request that everyone has respect. You can agree that everything you have read in this book has been suggestions, and in no way were you forced to believe anything. There have been multiple reminders to ensure that everyone has the freedom of choice.

Contrary to the unpopular belief among nonbelievers, everyone on this earth is considered a child of God. Yes, even murderers, abusers, or rapists are children of God. God knew that there would be a division among religions, and He knew that people would turn their backs on Him. God is okay with that, because He knows that each one of us will return to Him when the time is right. God will always love you, me, and everyone with an equal amount of love. I don't believe God has favorites. He actually proved that he loves everyone because he sacrificed his Son, Jesus Christ, to die for our sins. Take a moment to let that sink in. Jesus experienced so much pain on the cross. I believe that each wound that was caused by the nails piercing His skin, the swords in His sides, and the crown of thorns on His head, was equal to the sins that had been committed, that were being committed, and that would be committed. Jesus never complained about carrying a burden that he didn't have to. He did as his Father told him to do. If that is not love, then I don't know what is.

What Is the Purpose of Suffering?

Everyone has experienced some type of suffering, or they may have been affected in some way. Pain is something that we will experience every day. Pain and suffering don't wake up one morning and decide that today is a good day to hurt a couple of people. There is no bias about who yesterday's, today's, or tomorrow's targets are going to be. Something I have tried to understand is when I hear about children being diagnosed with incurable diseases or dying at the hands of others. I spoke to a lady who had been following a child on social media who had been diagnosed with a form of leukemia at the age of three months. He managed to have a successful bone marrow transplant, and everyone was over the moon with excitement.

The excitement was fleeting when he was diagnosed with grafts-versus-host disease (GvHD), which is the negative reaction of the body's immune system to the bone marrow transplant. The parents sold everything, and fundraising events were in full swing to get him the treatment he needed. Eventually, the family made it to Los Angeles, where the treatment for his GvHD started. Three years later, they left Los Angeles and went to Cincinnati for a different type of treatment. The little boy was responding well to the treatment, until another setback befell the family. The little boy had been diagnosed with skin cancer. Everyone was devastated, especially because the grandfather has also been diagnosed with skin cancer.

The grandfather passed away in 2020, and it was during this time that they received the news that they would have to leave the United States, because their medical visa had expired. Again, they had to pack up everything, and they flew to the United Kingdom. Mom, dad, and the two sisters were strong in their faith. They were asking for prayers for their beloved boy who was now a 13-year-old in a child's body. Sadly, the little boy lost his life to this terrible disease in 2021. His uncles and grandmother were angry. Every time someone told them that they were praying for them, someone would respond with a couple of expletive words that are not fit for any publication. The lady also told me that the grandmother had recently been diagnosed with cancer of the bladder.

I've heard many stories similar to this. I have read many posts where adults and children are facing life struggles and heartaches. Issues are not limited to one specific continent, country, town, county, village, or community. This is a daily occurrence that reaches each corner of this earth. The struggles, heartache, pain, and suffering are not limited to being diagnosed with a life-threatening illness, but also include natural weather disasters, financial hardships, injuries, abuse, and too many to mention here. Everyone wants to know why God is allowing these to happen. I know that people are going to kick their heels in when they see what I have to say, but take a couple of moments to reflect on what you are reading.

Humbleness

I remember an interaction between an elderly gentleman and his wife at the grocery store. He wanted to buy a bottle of wine, and his wife told him that he didn't need it and that it was bad for his health. He turned to her with a look of exasperation and told her that he was 88 years of age, his body wasn't his because he wouldn't be taking it with him, and that he should stop faffing because his soul was in tip-top shape. I knew she was swallowing back tears, because she squeaked when she apologized to him.

Did you know that you are not the owner of your body? I know, right? I was as shocked as you are when I found out that our bodies are on loan to us. We were trusted to take care of our rental property by treating it with the respect it deserves. The day you let out your last breath, your soul leaves your body and returns to heaven. The body you called yours will be returned to the earth by burial or cremation. Pain and suffering are constant reminders that we cannot control everything that happens in our lives. Would you like to hear another one of my little secrets? It's okay to relinquish the role of being the controller of your life and situations. I know that it is a frustrating task when things happen that you can't control, but it's all part of being humble. I can promise you that you won't crumble, you won't break, and you won't be a disappointment to anyone if you were to admit defeat. I would say that it would make you a very humble person.

Depending on God

- How many times have you begged, pleaded, and even bargained with God to heal someone you care about?

- How many times have you felt let down because your prayers aren't answered?

- How many times were you so angry at God because He didn't do as you demanded?

You would be holding up both hands with wriggling fingers, as well as both feet and wiggling toes. Secret time; God doesn't respond to begging, pleading, or bargaining tactics. What God wants from us is to be patient, and have faith. I have previously mentioned that human beings are impatient, and when we want something, we want it two weeks ago. God doesn't operate on threats, and His time moves differently than ours. You may feel as if you are being ignored and your prayers are not being answered, but you have to ask yourself the question: What are my motives for asking what I need or want? This is a question I can't answer for you, and neither can anyone else. As with many of the questions that I have asked, there are no right or wrong answers.

You have nothing to lose by putting a little more faith in God, and listening to or observing your surroundings for the answers you need. You never know who may enter your life, and you may never know why things happen the way they do. Not everything that happens is "in your face" or obvious, but do as I have constantly said throughout this book—keep an open mind.

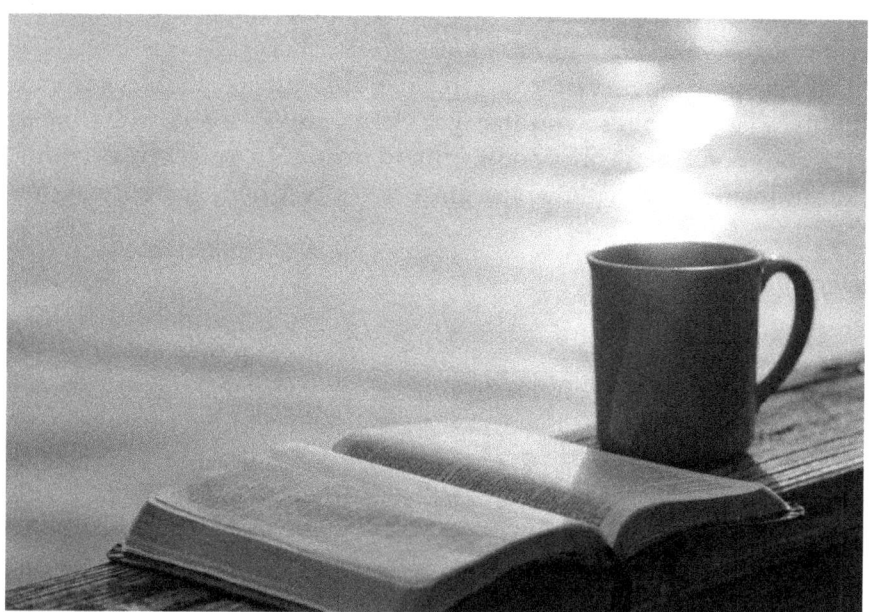

Roundup

The most important takeaway from the question of why God allows suffering is to remind us that earth is not a permanent place for us. We are on this earth to follow a destiny that is unknown to us. The pain and suffering we experience are a constant reminder to us of the pain that Jesus went through when He was crucified. Someone once told me that there is no such thing as a perfect person in a perfect world, and if you believe that everything is sunshine and roses, you would probably invest in new coloring pens. We have been conditioned to believe that everything has to be this way or that way, or that you have to look a certain way. We become so obsessed with perfection, that we have forgotten that we are perfect as we are. Genesis 1:27 says: "So God created mankind in His own image; in the image of God he created them; male and female he created them." Who are we to argue with the word of God? Do you need some more proof? Take a look at what Jeremiah 1:5 says: "Before I formed you in the womb I knew you, before you were born I set you apart; I appointed you as a prophet to the nations." Here is another one for good measure from Luke 12:6-7: "Are not five sparrows sold for two pennies? Yet not one of them is forgotten by God. Indeed, the very hairs of your head are all numbered. Don't be afraid; you are worth more than many sparrows."

You may feel as if you have been forgotten, neglected, or even forsaken by God—but you are loved and cherished. Learn to forgive yourself, and relinquish the anger and hurt you have burning inside of your soul. That is the biggest, most satisfying gift you can give yourself. I am going to end this chapter with something I heard years ago—Let go, and let God.

Chapter 9:

Start Over by Rediscovering Religion

I would like to invite you to bring your suitcase as you step foot on the last stop of our island-hopping cruise. This is the island where you can stroll around with your suitcase and its contents. Excuse me, what did you say? I didn't quite hear what you were saying. Oh, you don't have the suitcase anymore? I see, okay then. You say that you have a child's backpack? Of course, you are still welcome!

Are you one of those who has emptied their elephant-sized suitcase, and downgraded their luggage after each stop? Congratulations if you have. I would still like to congratulate you even if you haven't downgraded, because I know that you have had to face some very harrowing difficulties. You might not be in the place where you are ready to let go of everything, and that is perfectly fine. This journey has been as eye-opening for me, as I am sure it has been for you. I have found that whenever I start planning or writing a new book, I discover a little more about myself, or I find a piece of shrapnel that I didn't know was hiding inside me. You may have already noticed, but I am a very open-minded person. I welcome everyone into my world with open arms. Many of us know what it is like to be the odd one out. Many of us laughed with the bullies who mercilessly teased us, or avoided them because they had become vile in their bullying.

No one, but you, knows what your relationship with God or your deities is like. I'm not here to share my opinion on religion or spirituality with you, because that would be similar to shoving you into a corner. Would you have stuck around until now if I had been flinging all types of scriptures at you since the Introduction? No, you would not have, and I'm halfway positive that I would have jumped off the ship with you. I'm not here to convert your opinion about what religion or having a relationship with God is all about. However, I am here to share some information and stories about the experiences other people may have had. I've spoken to many people during my research, and everyone has an opinion about what religion means to them. Many even shared that they had been in a position where someone has tried to 'shove' the Bible down their throats. That is not me, and I don't care what others have to say. This book is about helping you break out of your invisible cage. I want you out of that cage, and living your life the way it is meant to be lived.

Finding the Right Path

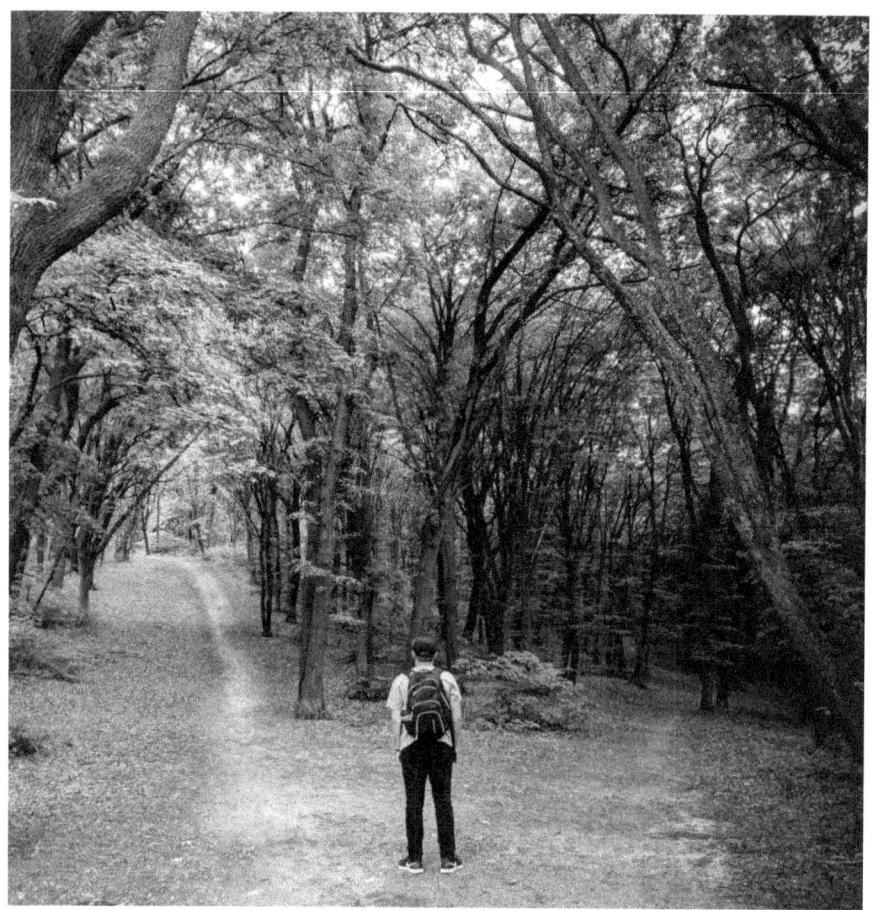

Imagine that you are standing at the intersection of a four-way crossroad. You are alone, and nobody is there to help you choose. The signboards that are meant to show you the direction have been ripped out of the ground. A mist of confusion, concern, fear, and panic is swirling around, because you don't know what to do. You will never know where each road will lead you, but you have to trust your gut instinct. Whichever direction you choose will be an adventure that you need to experience. I have seen many people standing at an intersection at some point during their lives. I have seen the agony they went through, because they were influenced by other's opinions. I can't even begin to tell you how many times I have wanted to be a buffer between the person making the choice and those telling what they should be doing.

Alex shared a story with me about their religious experience. They were at a crossroads in their religious journey. Alex had gone through a couple of difficult life changes in the space of three years. It was during these three years that Alex had a shift in their religious perspective. They refused to celebrate Easter or Christmas. When I asked why, they told me that a pastor had told them that Jesus Christ was not born on the 25th of December. They were told that Christmas was a Pagan holiday that came from the Catholic Church. Alex said that they would argue with everyone who dared force them to believe anything else.

This went on for close to nine years, and it wasn't until the world screeched to a halt because of a certain you-know-what inserted itself into our lives that she changed direction. Between the end of 2019 and the beginning of 2020, we had to adjust to the new normal. It was during this time that Alex had joined millions of others on the unemployment lines. Alex had always been a believer, but they admit that their views were skewed by a pastor who said one thing and acted based on another. Alex was listening to Christian music on YouTube when a recommendation popped up for a pastor in Singapore. They looked at it, dismissed it, and continued scrolling through YouTube—but something made them go back to this pastor. Alex clicked on the link to receive a notification when the church service would go live. That was the beginning of another life-altering moment for Alex.

They started following a pastor who presented the Bible in a way that they had never heard before. Alex says that they had never before left a sermon feeling as if the message was directed at them. They wanted more, and couldn't wait for the next sermon. When Christmas of 2020 started approaching, the pastor made a big deal about Christmas and let his followers know what an exciting time it was. He acknowledged that the 25th of December was not Jesus's actual birthday, but it was a universal date where everyone could take the day and remember its significance. Yes, Alex is still following the same pastor online, even though in-person services were due to start. The pastor had promised his followers, who are all across the globe, that he would continue to include them in his services.

Every Journey Starts Somewhere

Have you ever heard the story about the prodigal son? I would like to share a summarized version with you, because I believe that you may find comfort in this story. Please feel free to read the full text in Luke 15:11–31. This is a story about a father who had two sons. The father gave his sons their inheritance to do with what they wanted. The younger son, who initially asked for his inheritance, packed up and left to travel. He spent his money on everything, but had nothing to show for it. He found a job, but he didn't achieve the satisfaction he had hoped for, which was a plate of food. As one does when filled with jealousy or "what-ifs," the son started building up resentment toward his father and brother back at home. He imagined that they were thriving, had servants taking care of them, and were living in luxury, while he was fading away.

The younger son started his mission to return to the family estate, rehearsing his story about why he should be allowed to be welcomed back. He was willing to give up being a son, and would work as a servant. When the father saw his son, he ran to him and threw his arms around him as he welcomed him back with hugs and kisses. The son apologized for all that he had done, but the father did something that had both his sons gaping at him. The father called for a feast to be prepared to celebrate the return of the younger son. The older son was working in the fields when he heard the commotion. He went back to the house and asked his father what was going on, to which the father responded that his brother had returned.

This infuriated the older son, who refused to be part of the festivities. He was angry that he had worked his fingers to the bone, has been loyal to his father, and did everything that was required. He had never received any type of party from his father as a reward. His brother, on the other hand, had taken his money and wasted it—and when the river had run dry, he'd returned home. Luke 15:31–32 gives the son, and us, a response that lets us know how God feels about us: "My son," the father said, "you are always with me, and everything I have is yours. But we had to celebrate and be glad, because this brother of yours was dead and is alive again; he was lost and is found."

It doesn't matter how or where your new journey begins, as long as you start somewhere. You don't have to be afraid that you will not be welcomed back with open arms. I can't promise you a fattened calf, fireworks, or a party, but I can tell you that God will always welcome you back. He knew that you would find your way back when you set out on your own.

Helping You Overcome Obstacles

I have dropped enough breadcrumbs throughout our time together that I am confident that we could put together a couple of loaves of bread. Every single chapter has had something that you resonate with. You may not know what it is until you read it a couple of chapters later. The light bulb will go off, blinding you with understanding, and you realize that you may or may not be experiencing something similar. Is this some type of mind control tactic? The skeptics would love it if I said yes, but my answer to you—and everyone else who doubts my motives—is that I wouldn't know how to control anyone even if I tried.

This book has been about learning how to forgive the unforgivable. You are holding onto resentment, because you are afraid to let it go. You may be feeling powerful and in control when you have something to cling to. Others may be afraid to let go, because they fear that it may happen again. Many people may be harboring anger at God for not being there when they called for help. Have you perhaps thought that maybe God was there and you didn't notice because He didn't come in the way you thought He would? I want to share something that I shared previously, and if you hear it again, you might believe it. God will never forsake you, no matter what you think, or what you've been told. God is not a gambler, and He will never make any bets on your life.

Imagine that God and the devil are sitting side-by-side. They are watching you make a decision. God says, with the utmost confidence, that you are strong and you will make the right choice. The devil laughs, and says that you will fall into the temptation trap, and that you'll be his. God responds that it is okay if you do fall into the temptation trap, because it will be a learning experience for you, and that you will find your way back. The devil doesn't have a comeback.

God doesn't care whether we forgive Him or not, because he loves you regardless of how you feel. God loves every single person on this earth. He doesn't mind if we are angry at Him; because again, He knows that all paths lead right back to Him. God knows that when the time is right, we will seek Him out again, and He will be like the father welcoming his prodigal son. All we need to do is close our eyes and feel God's loving embrace. Still not too convinced you can forgive God for whatever reason? Let's take a look at some steps that may help you overcome obstacles that are preventing you from experiencing peace.

Taking Stock of Everything You Have

I am embarrassed to admit that I have been one of those who don't appreciate what I have. The whole world jumped on the "Air Fryer" bandwagon, and I wanted one, too. Social media platforms started sharing recipes, and everyone raved about the healthy food they were eating. I searched and compared prices, I looked at the different sizes, makes, and read the reviews. Rough calculations said that if I bought one, I would have to give up my morning coffee and biweekly donut for about two months. Then one has to weigh up the pros and cons about sizes, and make more calculations about which size would be best for the family; and I was just going around in never-ending circles until I stopped. I took stock of my kitchen. I have a stove, an oven, a microwave oven, and a toaster. My face started burning up because here I was, contemplating selling part of my liver to the highest bidder (giving up my morning coffee) to buy something that I already have.

From where I was standing, I knew that I was lucky because many people don't have half of what I have.

The moral of this story is that we get so blinded by our anger, hatred, fear, or sadness, that we don't see the beauty right before us. We should learn to stop living in the past, and concentrate on the here, and the now. We can't do anything about yesterday—no matter how much or how hard you try, you will not find what you lost or what was taken from you. You can be as angry as you want to be with God, but He will always love you. You can push Him as far as you want, but He will always be right beside you. You may feel as if you can't move through the jungle, but He will carry you.

Forgiveness and Trust

Why should you forgive God when I have said that He doesn't care? You are the person walking around on this earth, filled with whatever feelings that are preventing you from forgiving. Here's something you may know or have heard in passing—it all starts with you. You need to forgive yourself by unpacking everything you are holding back. I previously told you that Jesus died on the cross so that all our sins would be forgiven. Jesus died so that we didn't have to carry that burden. God loves us so much that he sacrificed his one and only Son, for you and me.

Trust is something that everyone struggles with, including me. I don't trust people, because I have been at the end where I have been burned one too many times. I told you, I'm an eternal optimist and I see good in everyone. While I may struggle with trusting my fellow human beings, there is one spiritual being I trust with everything—and yes, that is God. I know that He will come through for me when I need Him the most. He doesn't try to change me, but he fills me with the faith I need to carry me through the darkest hours. I have had so many people ask me why I would trust someone I can't see, touch, or hear. You should see the looks I get when I don't answer immediately, and a smile spreads across my face.

I see God in the beauty of the plants in my kitchen window, the new shoots of grass coming up after neglecting my garden, or even the beautiful blue skies. I see God when I look at myself in the mirror. Yes, I see God all around.

I can feel God when the wind blows against my skin or through my hair. I feel God when I stub my toes on the corner of my bed. I also feel God's hand on my head and heart when I'm sad, and the best feeling of all is when He tickles my insides to make me laugh. Oh yes, I can definitely feel God.

I can and have heard God. Everyone has their own version of what they hear. My experience has been that it is a voice I will never ignore. I was preparing a talk for a public speaking event, and my nerves were all over. I was shaking, the blood had drained from my body, and I was ready to back out and let someone else take over. Out of nowhere, I heard this voice boom through my head so clearly that I stopped and looked around the room: *Oh ye of little faith*! I took a couple of steps toward the master of ceremonies, and again; *Oh ye of little faith! Trust me, I'm here with you.* Well, who am I to argue with the voice in my head? I gave my talk with ease, the blood returned to my body, and I thanked God for the spiritual talking-to.

Love, Hope, and Faith

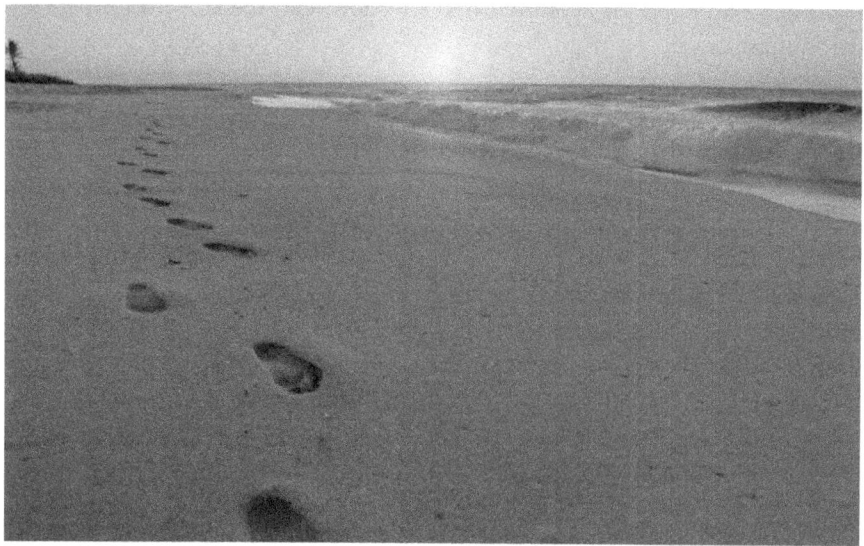

I would like to end this chapter with *Footprints In The Sand*. This is a poem that is special to me, and I believe that it summarizes us as people, and God's response to our doubt in Him. I'll see you on the last island.

One night a man had a dream. He dreamed he was walking along the beach with the Lord.

Across the sky flashed scenes from his life. For each scene he noticed two sets of footprints in the sand: one belonging to him, and the other to the Lord.

When the last scene of his life flashed before him, he looked back at the footprints in the sand.

He noticed that many times along the path of his life there was only one set of footprints.

He also noticed that it happened at the very lowest and saddest times in his life.

This really bothered him and he questioned the Lord about it:

"Lord, you said that once I decided to follow you, you'd walk with me all the way. But I have noticed that during the most troublesome times in my life, there is only one set of footprints. I don't understand why when I needed you most you would leave me."

The LORD replied:

"My son, my precious child, I love you and I would never leave you. During your times of trial and suffering, when you see only one set of footprints, it was then that I carried you." —Carolyn Joyce Carty

Conclusion

This must be my least favorite part of any book I write, and that is the Conclusion. I have two types of emotions that overwhelm me each time. I am excited to send you off with all the information, tool kits, and whatever else you may have learned throughout our time together. I am also sad, nervous, and anxious to let you go, because I worry about whether I have given you enough information to help you find your way through the jungle still holding you hostage. Am I a mother hen? Absolutely, without a shadow of a doubt. I don't like being an empty nester, because it gives me way too much time to think about what I could have done better to prepare you for what is waiting on the other end of this book.

We have reached the end of our island-hopping cruise together. I have to cut those apron strings, let you find your way through the jungle of life, and break out of your invisible cage. I am sending you off with the knowledge that I have equipped you with as much information as I could. Each chapter was written with the help of the caring hearts of others who have struggled to find their way through the good, the bad, and the ugly. The lessons learned may seem redundant and even repetitive, but they were inserted so that you would be reminded of the basics. I don't believe that it is necessary to run through everything that has been mentioned in this book, because we have dropped breadcrumbs all over. Thankfully, we don't have any birds cleaning up those breadcrumbs—you have got to love virtual tropical island cruises!

It's Okay Not to Be Okay

I want you to know, and it has been mentioned throughout this book—you don't have to do anything you aren't comfortable with. You have also learned that *YOU* can do whatever *YOU* need to help *YOU* improve *YOUR* life. I have inserted many gentle reminders, trigger warnings, and disclaimers where I felt it was applicable. I had to think about how I should end this cruise, without becoming all teary-eyed and causing a flood, and it came to me that I needed to send you off with some reassurance. I believe that this is an excellent parting note as you gather your elephant-sized, regular, or small suitcase, backpack, or purse as you prepare to disembark from the ship.

You need to know that you don't need anyone's approval about what you should or should not be doing. There is absolutely no shame whatsoever in seeking professional help. I have found that people are afraid to get professional help, because it will make them seem weak. Don't allow those from different faiths, religions, or backgrounds to influence you with their opinions. You know that the one-size-fits-all label on clothing is a myth, and the same applies when it comes to seeking therapy or professional help. You need to do what you feel is right, and not what your friend's aunt's grocer's hairdresser's grandfather's roommate in the nursing home tells you is right. Remember that this is your life, your body, and your mind. Okay, technically it's not your body, but you know what I mean—settle down skeptics.

Hearty Reassurances

I know, that you know, that it's okay not to be okay. I also know that the little doubt bubble is bouncing around from side to side, because it has a job to do. You have more power than you think over that doubt bubble—so yes, you are in control of it. My parting gift to you is the gift of hearty reassurances to reaffirm that you will be okay. March to the beat of your own drums, and don't ever give anyone a sliver of a gap to steal your happiness. Be who you are, and who you are meant to be. Be the strong and courageous person who is stepping out of the invisible cage that held you captive for way too long.

- Don't settle for anything less than the best.

- Reach out to someone who can lead you in the right direction.

- It's okay to break down; it's not a sign of weakness when cracks start appearing.

- You are not made of clay, porcelain, or glass; you too will break when you aren't treated well.

- Take as long as you need to find what it is you need.

- Have faith in your strength.

- If and when you are ready, start a conversation with your deity of choice; a simple hello is all that you need to open the line of communication.

- Don't be too hard on yourself; you don't want to undo all the positive work you have already achieved.

- Help is just around the corner.

- You are a precious commodity to everyone you touch with your words, smiles, voice, or tears.

Until We Meet Again: Thank you, and See You Later

Thank you, again, for joining me on this cruise. I have learned so much more about myself in the process. The world you live in is beautiful, bright, and full of life because you add your flair and character. You are the keeper of your world, and you have what it takes to keep it away from the shadows that threaten your happiness. Never let anyone tell you that you don't deserve happiness, because it is a blatant lie. I hope that I've helped you realize your worth and place in this world, even if it was repeated after someone else told you. You may be skeptical, but don't join the skeptics who want to find fault in everything. Believe, have faith, and know that you can and will do anything to benefit your mental, physical, and emotional health and well-being.

The cruise may be ending, but I would like to let you know that you will always have me in the palm of your hand. You will always be welcome whenever you need a nonjudgmental, and condemnation-free safe place. May I ask that you please consider leaving a review after you have completed the cruise, and share your experience with me, and everyone else so that everyone will know that they aren't alone on this crazy journey through the jungles of the tropical islands. Please remember to be kind to yourself, and heed Maya Angelou's advice as shared as you read the last words on your way out.

It's one of the greatest gifts you can give yourself, to forgive. Forgive everybody. — Maya Angelou

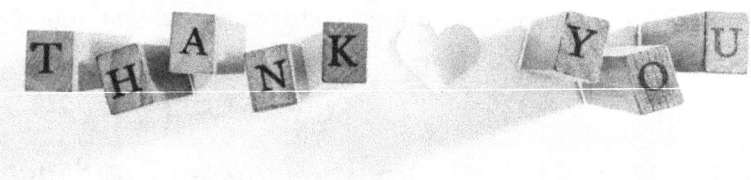

References

The ancient Hawaiian practice of forgiveness. (2018). Uplift. https://uplift.love/the-ancient-hawaiian-practice-of-forgiveness

Ballenger, M. (2019, September 5). *3 Reasons God is allowing you to emotionally suffer*. Apply Gods Word. https://applygodsword.com/3-reasons-god-is-allowing-you-to-emotionally-suffer

Bissell, J. (2019, August 12). *8 Ways to learn how to forgive rather than hold a grudge, according to experts*. Bustle. https://www.bustle.com/p/how-to-forgive-not-hold-a-grudge-18649034

Blundell, A. (2019). *Healthy boundaries — 12 Signs you lack them (And why you need them)*. Harley Therapy Blog. https://www.harleytherapy.co.uk/counselling/healthy-boundaries.htm

Breese, I. (2020, May 7). *The ultimate path to healing, what to do if you're angry, even at God*. Medium. https://medium.com/publishous/the-ultimate-path-to-healing-even-if-youre-angry-at-god-e2ab80709451

Brown, M. (2017, March 16). *5 Reasons that God allows suffering*. South Bay Bible Church. https://www.southbaychurchli.org/life-purpose-hope-blog/5-reasons-that-god-allows-suffering

Bufkin, G. (2017, February 18). *Why does God allow pain?*. Home of Grace Faith-Based Addiction Recovery. https://www.homeofgrace.org/blog/why-does-god-allow-pain-hint-its-one-of-his-greatest-blessings

Campbell, L. (2021, June 7). *Why personal boundaries are important and how to set them*. Psych Central. https://psychcentral.com/lib/what-are-personal-boundaries-how-do-i-get-some

Cleveland Clinic. (2021, December 10). *Cortisol*. My.clevelandclinic.org. https://my.clevelandclinic.org/health/articles/22187-cortisol

Domonell, K. (2017, October 9). *6 Ways stress is hurting your health—And what you can do about it*. Right as Rain by UW Medicine. https://rightasrain.uwmedicine.org/mind/stress/6-ways-stress-hurting-your-health-and-what-you-can-do-about-it

The Editors. (2021, May 30). *How to forgive someone who hurt you emotionally*. Upjourney. https://upjourney.com/how-to-forgive-someone-who-hurt-you-emotionally

Enright, R. (2015, October 15). *Eight keys to forgiveness*. Greater Good. https://greatergood.berkeley.edu/article/item/eight_keys_to_forgiveness

Fisher, A. (2022, April 17). *How to stop holding a grudge and move on*. Psych Central. https://psychcentral.com/health/tips-to-stop-holding-a-grudge

Footprints in the sand poem. (n.d.). Scrapbook. https://www.scrapbook.com/poems/doc/38987.html

Frankish, F. (2022, February 11). *10 Ways to respond when someone hurts you deeply*. Hack Spirit. https://hackspirit.com/when-someone-hurts-you-deeply

Goodreads. (n.d.). *A quote by Gloria Tesch*. Goodreads.com. https://www.goodreads.com/quotes/601979-there-is-a-time-and-place-for-everything-you-just

Harrison, P. (2021, January 11). *Forgiveness meditation script to help you let go*. The Daily Meditation. https://www.thedailymeditation.com/forgiveness

Healey, J. (2019, July 23). *Ho'oponopono prayer for forgiveness, healing and making things right*. Healing Brave.

https://healingbrave.com/blogs/all/hooponopono-prayer-for-forgiveness

Holtz, J. (2022, March 3). *Mindfulness meditation can reduce guilt, leading to unintended negative social consequences.* UW News. https://www.washington.edu/news/2022/03/03/mindfulness-meditation-can-reduce-guilt-leading-to-unintended-negative-social-consequences

Holub, A. (2014, December 3). *13 Health benefits of forgiveness.* WisdomTimes. https://www.wisdomtimes.com/blog/health-benefits-of-forgiveness

How to cope with traumatic stress. (2021). American Psychological Association. https://www.apa.org/topics/trauma/stress

How to let go of a grudge. (2019, August 22). Modern Therapy. https://moderntherapy.online/blog-2/2019/8/22/how-to-let-go-of-a-grudge

James, M. (2011, May 23). *The Hawaiian secret of forgiveness.* Psychology Today. https://www.psychologytoday.com/us/blog/focus-forgiveness/201105/the-hawaiian-secret-forgiveness

Joseph, D. I. (n.d.). *Why does God allow pain? (Biblical reasons explained).* Christianity FAQ. https://christianityfaq.com/why-does-god-allow-pain

Martin, S. (2017, March 5). *Benefits of setting boundaries: Why you need to set healthy boundaries.* Live Well with Sharon Martin. https://www.livewellwithsharonmartin.com/6-benefits-of-setting-boundaries

Martin, S. (2021). *What kind of boundaries do you need to set?.* The Better Boundaries Workbook. https://betterboundariesworkbook.com/types-of-boundaries

Maya Angelou quotes. (n.d.). BrainyQuote. https://www.brainyquote.com/quotes/maya_angelou_578747

Mayo Clinic Staff. (2020, November 13). *Forgiveness: Letting go of grudges and bitterness.* Mayo Clinic. https://www.mayoclinic.org/healthy-lifestyle/adult-health/in-depth/forgiveness/art-20047692

Mayo Clinic Staff. (2022, April 29). *Meditation: A simple, fast way to reduce stress.* Mayo Clinic. https://www.mayoclinic.org/tests-procedures/meditation/in-depth/meditation/art-20045858

Mental Health CTR. (2021, January 22). *Trauma focused therapy for adults.* MentalHealthCTR.com. https://www.mentalhealthctr.com/trauma-focused-therapy-for-adults

Merriam-Webster. (n.d.). Forgive. In *Merriam-Webster.com dictionary.* Retrieved June 7, 2022, from https://www.merriam-webster.com/dictionary/forgive

The National Child Traumatic Stress Network. (2018). *Trauma types.* Nctsn.org. https://www.nctsn.org/what-is-child-trauma/trauma-types

Negroni, J. (2013, December 10). *7 Steps to true forgiveness.* Thriveworks. https://thriveworks.com/blog/7-steps-to-true-forgiveness

New International Version. (1993). BibleGateway.com. https://www.biblegateway.com/passage/?search=luke+23%3A34&version=NIV

A quote by Gloria Tesch. (n.d.). Goodreads. https://www.goodreads.com/quotes/601979-there-is-a-time-and-place-for-everything-you-just

A quote by Robert Muller. (n.d.). Goodreads. https://www.goodreads.com/quotes/113417-to-forgive-is-the-highest-most-beautiful-form-of-love

Rebecca. (2020, June 10). *How to let go of the past: 15 Powerful steps to take.* Minimalism Made Simple. https://www.minimalismmadesimple.com/home/let-go-of-the-past

Rees, M. (2018, March 27). *How grudges hold you back from happiness (And how to forgive)*. Whole Life Challenge. https://www.wholelifechallenge.com/how-grudges-hold-you-back-from-happiness-and-how-to-forgive

Rom, M. (2016, September 6). *An ancient Hawaiian practice for forgiveness*. Meredith Rom. https://www.meredithrom.com/blog-articles/2016/8/8/an-ancient-hawaiian-practice-for-forgiveness

Schumacker, L. (2019, April 14). *8 Signs you're holding a grudge even if you don't think you are*. Insider. https://www.insider.com/signs-you-are-holding-grudge-2019-4

Smith, M., & Robinson, L. (2021a, November). *Helping someone with PTSD*. HelpGuide. https://www.helpguide.org/articles/ptsd-trauma/helping-someone-with-ptsd.htm

Smith, M., Robinson, L., & Segal, J. (2021b, November). *How to cope with traumatic events*. HelpGuide. https://www.helpguide.org/articles/ptsd-trauma/traumatic-stress.htm

Star, K. (2021, November 11). *Learning how to forgive when you have anxiety*. Verywell Mind. https://www.verywellmind.com/learning-to-forgive-2584075

Thurmond, N. (2019). *Healing from trauma and setting boundaries in relationships*. Eating Disorder Hope. https://www.eatingdisorderhope.com/treatment-for-eating-disorders/co-occurring-dual-diagnosis/trauma-ptsd/healing-from-trauma-and-setting-boundaries-in-relationships

USA TODAY. (2018, January 8). *Mom comes face-to-face with her son's killer in court* [Video]. YouTube. https://www.youtube.com/watch?v=0Z5SGI5Jdns

Vanbuskirk, S. (2021, August 19). *The mental health effects of holding a grudge*. Verywell Mind. https://www.verywellmind.com/the-mental-health-effects-of-holding-a-grudge-5176186

Image References

Babienko, V. (2018, June 15). *Man at the crossroads*. [Image]. Unsplash. https://unsplash.com/photos/KTpSVEcU0XU

Bradshaw, R. (2020, June 21). *Turning point and dead end road sign*. [Image]. Unsplash. https://unsplash.com/photos/1PPoNhMzAmY

Burden, A. (2017, April 12). [*Green ceramic mug beside book*]. [Image]. Unsplash. https://unsplash.com/photos/4eWwSxaDhe4

Canty, J. (2020, August 14). *A very foggy morning on my friend's farm near Chehalis, Washington. He had many horses and was always checking his fence for damage*. [Image]. Unsplash. https://unsplash.com/photos/eZtLqACNlbM

Chouette, L. (2021, April 14). [*White and pink flower on white textile*]. [Image]. Unsplash. https://unsplash.com/photos/xsx1pgVmnjw

Cornish, F. (2018, February 10). *Fairy bonsai*. [Image]. Unsplash. https://unsplash.com/photos/Uq3gTiPlqRo

Hedger, C. (2017, August 10). *Thank you wooden cubes*. [Image]. Unsplash. https://unsplash.com/photos/t48eHCSCnds

iMattSmart. (2020, April 14). *Unlocked old fashioned padlock. Just when will lockdown end?*. [Image]. Unsplash. https://unsplash.com/photos/Vp3oWLsPOss

Kaleidico. (2018, July 26). [*Two people drawing on whiteboard*]. [Image]. Unsplash. https://unsplash.com/photos/26MJGnCM0Wc

Leonhardt, N. (2020, March 15). *Long exposure capture of Phinizy Swamp, Augusta, Georgia, USA. Visit my website: nilsleonhardt.com*. [Image]. Unsplash. https://unsplash.com/photos/Tss1uOMczDg

Luther, C. (2021, August 9). [*Red and black cap on brown wooden chest box*]. [Image]. Unsplash. https://unsplash.com/photos/e0l5ty0oY1M

Reyes, A. (2019, April 2). [*White cruise ship under cloudy sky*]. [Image]. Unsplash. https://unsplash.com/photos/LWFdBz4d6nE

Saidi, H. (2021, January 2). [*Black and white wooden signage*]. [Image]. Unsplash. https://unsplash.com/photos/9cgMKmZyhH0

Schneider, P. (2018, September 3). [*Woman sitting on sand field*]. [Image]. Unsplash. https://unsplash.com/photos/yw1y-alKGrg

Simonides, M. (2021, April 27). *A fully laden Volga whizzes by*. [Image]. Unsplash. https://unsplash.com/photos/GYZ9F3U1gBk

Spiske, M. (2019, March 15). *Made with Canon 5d Mark III and Meyer Optik Görlitz Primoplan 1.9 / 75mm*. [Image]. Unsplash. https://unsplash.com/photos/wcAOi6t0qaA

Thejus, T. (2020, January 6). *This pic was shot during pre wedding shoot of my cousin around afternoon with clear sky and sunny outdoors*. [Image]. Unsplash. https://unsplash.com/photos/0OEO1M41R1I

Wilkinson, S. (2021, May 3). *Abuse. Ongoing trauma. Low self-esteem. Boxed in by pain. Fragile hearts, broken and darkened*. [Image]. Unsplash. https://unsplash.com/photos/EDJKEXFbzHA

Wong, J. (2020, December 5). *Footsteps in the sand during sunrise*. [Image]. Unsplash. https://unsplash.com/photos/DcdwkU35IW0

Wright, K. (2019, February 8). *Believe in yourself*. [Image]. Unsplash. https://unsplash.com/photos/yMg_SMqfoRU

www.ingramcontent.com/pod-product-compliance
Lightning Source LLC
Chambersburg PA
CBHW050319010526
44107CB00055B/2314